Jesse Cannone

THE END OF
ALL DISEASE

Simple, Little-Known,
and Proven Cures
for 7 of the Most
Dangerous Diseases

Disclaimer

The information in this book is provided for informational purposes only and is not a substitute for professional medical advice. The author and publisher make no legal claims, express or implied, and the material is not intended to replace the services of a physician.

The author, publisher and/or copyright holder assume no responsibility for any loss or damage caused, or allegedly caused, directly or indirectly by the use of the information contained in this book. The author and publisher specifically disclaim any liability incurred from the use or application of the contents of this book.

All rights reserved. No part of this book may be reproduced or transmitted in any form or by any means, electronic, mechanical, photocopying, recording or otherwise, without the prior written permission of the publisher.

This book shares and interprets the research and discoveries of several medical professionals. This information was gathered through interviews and articles written for the Healthy Back Institute and Live Pain Free newsletter or from publicly available sources. Credit has been given to those experts for their intellectual property, and this book is simply relaying the information shared by them with readers, making no claims contrary to the existing copyrighted works of these experts.

Throughout this book, trademarked names are referenced. Rather than putting a trademark symbol in every occurrence of a trademarked name, we state that we are using the names in an editorial fashion only and to the benefit of the trademark owner with no intention of infringement of the trademark.

Published by the Healthy Back Institute
141 E. Mercer Street, Suite E
Dripping Springs, TX 78620
1 (800) 216-4908

Dedication

This book is for *you*. You are tired of giving control of your health and happiness to someone else. *You* know that you deserve better than the medical treatment and lies that still leave you suffering. This book will show you a better way—a way to bring yourself out of the depths of your pain and suffering, to the light at the end of the tunnel. A future of wellness is within your reach.

Acknowledgments

This book is the culmination of years of my personal quest to find the real, proven cures for the world's common ailments. You may be reading my words, but I am forever in the debt of the answers I found, and the experts who shared those answers with me. I could not have put this book together without the support, guidance, information, help, and honest feedback of countless others.

I'd like to thank the dozens of doctors and experts I interviewed, or whose work I studied, for their time and information as I researched the various aspects of the diseases and cures in this book. These experts include: Kathleen Barnes, Dr. David Berceli, Dr. Hal Blatman, John G. Bruhn, Dr. Stanislaw Burzynski, Dr. Ignacio Chamorro Balda, Dr. Hulda Clark, Amber Davies, Dr. Greg Fors, Vivian Goldschmidt, Dr. Nicholas J. Gonzalez, Dr. Frank Lawlis, Dr. Dwight Lundell, Dr. Jim Maas, Dr. Jim Oschman, Dr. Maggie Phillips, Dr. John Sarno, Dr. Frank Shallenberger, Dr. Robert Thompson, Dr. Mark Wiley, and Stewart Wolf.

In addition to these pioneers and experts, many others have contributed to my knowledge of the body, mind, and diet. I've done my best to pass as much of the information they taught me on to you.

This book could not have come together without the tireless efforts of Helen Chang, Kristine Serio, and the Author Bridge Media team. They spent countless hours assisting me with planning and editing the contents of this book into the polished form you see today.

Table of Contents

INTRODUCTION:

The Path to Wellness

The Crisis of Modern Health

Good health is one of the most precious things we have. Without our health, the rest of life slips away from us. We can't do the things we want to do or appreciate the opportunities that come our way each day. Vitality, productivity, strength, joy—all of these and more are built on a foundation of good health.

Health is so fundamental to our well-being that you would think the health system in the United States—one of the most advanced countries in the world—would be top notch. On the surface, that even seems to be the case. The US spent approximately $3.8 trillion on health care in 2013, according to one estimate by *Forbes*—almost twice as much per capita as the next-highest spender on the list. Yet the Commonwealth Fund ranked us last in a health care study of eleven developed countries. How can that be possible?

It's possible because medicine in the US isn't about health. It's about disease.

Think about this for a minute. What happens when you get sick? You go to your primary care physician, and you present your signs and symptoms: "I have a pain in my head," or "I've been getting a lot of cramps." Your physician then takes that information and diagnoses it. "You have chronic migraines," or "You have irritable bowel syndrome."

Then, once your symptoms have a label, the physician treats that label. And the treatment most always involves at least one kind of drug, and sometimes more.

This is a failed model of treatment. It's also a sad reality.

Most physicians are looking at and trying to treat your disease itself. They're not looking at the underlying *cause* of the disease. By treating the signs and symptoms of the disease—the pain, the discomfort, the sweating, the nausea—they are just fixing the results. They rarely step back and evaluate you and your symptoms as an entire person.

By zooming in and focusing only on the effects of the problem, they miss the bigger picture. They don't consider that your mind, your body, and your diet all work together to bring you sickness or health.

They're not focused on bringing your body back to wellness. And they're even less focused on helping you understand how you can avoid the same situation in the future.

The average person trusts their doctor to know how to diagnose health problems, and how to prescribe medicines and procedures to fix them. But the scary truth is that, much of the time, even doctors are basing their diagnosis and treatment at least as much on medical *belief* as medical knowledge. That's what they were taught to do in medical school and during their internships and residencies. And that's what they'll probably keep learning to do. Why?

Because the professors and doctors writing the medical textbooks don't know, don't believe, or don't want to believe the truth about whole-body balance. They just want to look for a simple cause-and-effect scenario, where one symptom is treated by one drug. And it just doesn't work that way.

Beyond all that, an equally if not more serious problem complicating why the medical establishment hasn't yet embraced new, cutting-edge therapies is this: simple economics.

The medical profession is a business. And like people in any business, all parties involved have a major stake in protecting their incomes: doctors, insurance companies, pharmaceutical companies—everyone except you, the patient. For years, drug companies have been one of the biggest sources of money pouring into this industry. So why is there an incentive to research natural products? Why is there an incentive to find a cure or treatment that doesn't involve a drug?

There is no incentive. And the sad fact is that the more sick people there are, the more business this so-called "health care" model generates.

Not everyone in the medical profession is out to put profits above all else. Many people are caught in the system and just can't break out. Others aren't fully aware of the situation. And some people are even fighting to break the mold. But at the end of the day, profits and corporate concerns are still dominating the industry, while the health of the nation suffers.

Medicine is sacrificing its sense of compassion in the name of corporate greed.

Something needs to change. Fortunately, thanks to the efforts of modern wellness pioneers, the revolution has already begun.

Wellness Pioneer

What if I told you that 80 percent of what people believe about good health is wrong, and the 20 percent of people who are called "quacks" and "crazy" are actually right?

My name is Jesse Cannone, and I have helped hundreds of thousands of people to reclaim a high quality of life based on the fundamental wellness methods I'll share with you in this book. I am the cofounder of the Healthy Back Institute and one of the leading back pain experts in the world. I've helped people in more than 120 countries to relieve or eliminate debilitating back pain, and that number grows every day.

I've been featured as an expert in dozens of newspapers and magazines, including *Men's Fitness, Balance, The Washington Examiner,* and *Women's World.* I have also appeared numerous times on television and radio programs, including NBC and MSNBC, and I am the author of *The 7 Day Back Pain Cure,* as well as the editor-in-chief of the *Live Pain Free* subscription newsletter.

I've spent my career searching out the world's leading medical and wellness pioneers to expand my knowledge of alternative and holistic health methods that mainstream Western medicine is trying to keep under the rug. In this book, I'll share that knowledge with you and show you how to take your health into your own hands, where it truly belongs.

Your Health, in Your Hands

We're at a point in time where our entire body of scientific knowledge and technology is revolutionized every two to three years. And yet it takes the medical establishment closer to seventeen years to embrace and adopt new findings, and to implement these findings into standardized care.

Traditional medicine is failing to keep up with the pace of scientific advancement. That means that if you are suffering from pain or disease, you are missing out on solutions that can restore your health and transform your life.

The End of All Disease is designed to change all that. This book pulls together my decades of expertise and the combined research of the most knowledgeable health experts on the front lines of health and wellness today. The information and strategies in these pages will revolutionize the way you approach your health. They will change your understanding of how wellness works and show you how you can use these simple yet powerful principles to end your pain and disease for good.

If you are looking for the path to true wellness, you've found it.

You and I will take this journey together. We'll uncover the little-known secrets to health and wellness; then we'll use them to create new balance in your health and in your life. From this foundation, you'll learn the cures to seven of the worst diseases in the world today. More than that, you'll also gain the knowledge and power to take control of your health, regardless of your situation, symptoms, or conditions.

The time to take your health into your own hands is now. Your true path to wellness starts in one place: with the Wellness Model of Health™. I'll take you on the first step of this revolutionary system in chapter 1.

Your journey to health starts now.

PART I:

The Foundation of Healthy, Pain-Free Living

CHAPTER 1:

The Wellness Model of Health

The Wellness Model of Health™

When was the last time you saw your doctor because you felt well?

For most of us, the answer to that question is probably "never." That's because mainstream Western medicine is based on a disease model of health.

Our health care system is focused on treating the symptoms of disease. Think about it. How many doctors have you seen who asked you what your symptoms were, wrote you a prescription for a drug, and sent you on your way? Unless you're in the extreme minority, you've probably never met a doctor who handled your problem any other way.

Now imagine that something else happened when you went in for your doctor's visit. It starts in the usual way. Your doctor asks you all the common questions about your symptoms, when they started, and if it's happened before. But then, instead of pulling out the prescription pad . . . the conversation continues.

You're asked about what foods you eat regularly, how much water you drink, and if you take supplements. You find yourself answering questions about how you deal with stressful situations and if you take enough time to recharge your emotions. You start to tell your doctor about more than just your body's symptoms; you answer questions about your mind and diet as well.

By the time you walk out of that office, instead of a prescription for a liver-killing pain drug in your hand, you leave with a strategy to eliminate certain foods from your diet, an exercise plan, and a set of recommendations to restore balance to your overall health. Instead of being told to eliminate salt from your diet and swallow a statin drug every morning, you have a plan to improve your health without taking a single drug.

This is what a visit to the doctor *should* be like. When doctors and patients have the knowledge to identify the true causes behind disease and come up with solutions that treat the entire person, that person can get on a path to wellness.

Unfortunately, most of us will never get that level of treatment. Doctors can't give what they aren't taught, professors can't teach what they don't know, and drug companies won't share what they can't sell.

We can't continue on with this destructive pattern. Too much of our happiness and joy in life depends on good health. Not the Band-Aid of suppressed disease symptoms, but real health that comes from the inside out. Our disease-focused health paradigm needs to change. And the way to change it is with the Wellness Model of Health™.

The Wellness Model of Health™ treats the cause of your pain or illness. It's a completely different approach than what you're used to. In this model, you do look at the physical signs and symptoms you have, but you don't stop there. You take it deeper. You figure out why your body is out of balance in the first place, and you look into how to reestablish your overall balance to restore optimal health.

True health is about free flow. It's about returning yourself to your natural state of peak physical and mental harmony. This is the Wellness Model of Health™, and right here, right now, it is within your reach, starting with its foundation: the Complete Healing Formula™.

The Complete Healing Formula™: Mind, Body, Diet

Your health has three key areas: mind, body, and diet. If you want to achieve true wellness, then you need to address all three of these. When you create balance in all three areas, you have achieved what I call the Complete Healing Formula™.

The Complete Healing Formula™ is the engine of the Wellness Model of Health™. Understanding how your mind, body, and diet work together to bring you true health is the starting point for real recovery. Let's look at each of these in detail.

Your Mind

Your mind is the first piece of the Complete Healing Formula™, and it plays a powerful role in your health.

First, I want to assure you that when I talk about the mind, I'm not saying that "the pain is all in your head." Your physical pain is real. But your beliefs and your attitude toward your condition can have a huge impact on your body's ability to recover and heal. Your mental willingness to participate in any particular treatment can help you achieve the level of wellness you're looking for.

And it doesn't stop there. Your mindset about your life and the world in general can also have a big impact on your overall health. People with positive states of mind tend to overcome obstacles, injuries, and diseases much faster than people who have negative states of mind.

No one argues that the mind can have an impact on our physical bodies. Just recall a time you were frightened and the speed of your breathing increased, or you started sweating. Or maybe you were watching a tragic movie and before you knew it, you found yourself crying. In both of these examples, your mind triggered a physical response in your body. In a similar way, your health is affected by your emotions, beliefs, and levels of stress.

For example, Dr. John E. Sarno, a pioneer in the treatment of back pain, talks about the concept of Tension Myositis Syndrome (TMS), or mind-body syndrome. When something in your life causes you to feel a negative emotion, you experience mild oxygen deprivation in your body. This oxygen deprivation can lead to muscle spasms, swelling joints, and aches. Your mental stress creates a physical problem. Best-selling author Louise Hay has also been showing us the correlation between physical problems and mental thought patterns for over thirty years, beginning with her book, *Heal Your Body*.

Our minds and our bodies are undeniably connected. The sooner we can get them to work in harmony together, the healthier we'll be. I'll talk more about the power of your mind in later chapters.

Your Body

The second of the three areas of health is your body, and it of course also plays a critical role in the Complete Healing Formula™.

The body is the main thing people look at when they're ill or in pain. Earlier, I talked about how the modern health paradigm runs into problems because it focuses so exclusively on the body. But the problem runs deeper than that.

Even when they look at the body, most modern health professionals only consider a specific part of it when they target a problem. Let's say that you have back pain. You go to your doctor, who gives you a prescription for an anti-inflammatory drug. You take the drug, and it gives you temporary relief by masking the pain—but at a price. Beyond failing to address the underlying cause of the problem, that drug is dangerous to other parts of your body.

Or you visit your chiropractor, and he says that your spine is out of alignment. He manipulates the spine back into place, but again, the results are only temporary. That's why most people have to go back to their chiropractor one or two times a week. The chiropractor is only targeting one specific part of your body. The spinal misalignment you have isn't isolated. It's caused by muscle imbalances. Your bones go where your muscles pull them. If you don't address why your bones are out of alignment in the first place, you're going to find yourself going around in circles.

High cholesterol is another example. Doctors commonly advise you to reduce your cholesterol by prescribing a statin drug. The drug alters the way the body naturally functions in order to knock down your cholesterol number—something in itself that most doctors are misinformed about and that can actually be dangerous, as I'll cover later. Regardless, when you isolate your cholesterol from other important health factors and neglect the reasons that your cholesterol is high to begin with, you won't see any lasting change to your health.

To be clear, I'm not saying you should stop going to the doctor. I'm not saying you should stop doing chiropractic care. What I want you to do is look at all the pieces of the puzzle so that you can get the best results from your different treatments.

When you're looking at your body, you have to be aware of all aspects of it, and how they work together to support your health.

Your Diet

The third key part of the three areas of health and the Complete Healing Formula™ is your diet. Most people don't realize that your diet plays an enormous role not just in how much you weigh or how you feel, but also in whether you have pain and are able to heal quickly.

Most of us don't eat very well to begin with. And even when we do, we don't get enough vitamins, minerals, and antioxidants. We get too much junk, chemicals, preservatives, and toxins in our food and water. Even if you do eat well, there are still certain things you need to be healthy that you won't get in your diet. I'll go into detail about how you can begin to build a healthy diet in later chapters.

Diet is just as important to the Complete Healing Formula™ as mind and body, but again, it won't take care of your pain and illness on its own. You have to address all three areas. The three of them come together to form your health as a whole person. For example, when your mind and body are under stress, you need more caloric energy from quality vitamins, minerals, and nutrients to help you heal and repair.

It's critical to be aware of your diet and the way it works with your mind and body to play its part in your pain and healing.

The Three Hidden Causes of All Health Conditions

The Complete Healing Formula™ gives you the foundation you need to rebuild your wellness. Next, I want to introduce to you to the second half of the Wellness Model of Health™; the tools that will make that rebuilding possible.

There are three hidden causes of all health conditions: excess, deficiencies, and stagnation. This model was pioneered and developed by Dr. Mark Wiley in the late 1990s while he was traveling around Asia meeting with shamans, healers, bonesetters, herbalists and other traditional medicine men in search of the key to optimal wellness, and it makes a lot of sense.

I'll begin with terms that are slightly technical, and then explain what they mean in plain English. Once you understand these key concepts, you'll probably never look at your own pain or illness the same way again.

Let's start where your health *should* be: at homeostasis. As Dr. Wiley points out in his book, *Arthritis Reversed,* homeostasis is the body's baseline of health and well-being. It is the state where you feel good—not too stressed, tired, or excited. You are in a state where your digestion is working properly, your body is absorbing proper amounts of nutrients, and oxygen and is expelling toxins through the skin, lungs, and intestines. Your sleep and wake cycle is set, you work and exercise, you have a balanced home-work-social life. Things are good.

But life often gets in the way and we don't feel as good anymore. Poor health, pain, and disease are all felt in the body (or mind) when it is off balance or is no longer functioning at homeostasis. In that case, what is the bottom line of health?

All pain and disease is ultimately caused by one (or more) of the following three issues:

1. Excess ("too much")

2. Deficiency ("too little")

3. Stagnation ("too slow")

All these terms revolve around one idea: that to live in optimal health, free from pain, you need to maintain a delicate balance in your body, mind, and diet.

Beyond Your Body

When you address your excesses, deficiencies, and stagnations across all three facets of mind, body, and diet, you create your personal Wellness Model of Health™, fueled by the Complete Healing Formula™.

This is a key concept. It's not just about your mental outlook. It's not just about physical therapy and anti-inflammatory medications. It's not just about what you eat every day. All of those things are critically important, and they all need to be addressed as key factors on your journey to optimal wellness.

You need to keep an eye out for excess, deficiency, and stagnation—not just in your body, but in your mind and diet as well. It's important to avoid too much (i.e., excess) of anything that causes you pain, or too little (i.e., deficiency) of something in order to prevent pain or illness from occurring. Excess, deficiency, or stagnation in even one of these three key areas can harm your health and overall wellness.

In fact, most if not all health problems are the direct result of imbalances in your body, mind, and diet. So let's look at the three concepts of excess, deficiency, and stagnation in more detail to help you figure out where you could be going wrong.

Excess: Too Much of Something

When I talk about excess, I'm talking about too much of something. Often we think of our diet when we consider excesses related to poor health, such as too much sugar, too much cholesterol, or too much salt (two of which are actually myths, by the way, as I'll cover in later chapters). We can also have excesses in our bodies or minds, such as inflammation or stress. In all cases, excessive amounts of something will lead to problems. Here are a few examples.

If you drink too much soda, coffee, or caffeinated drinks, you'll have too much caffeine (excess) in your system (as well as other junk). Since caffeine is a diuretic that causes you to urinate a lot, you'll have too little water (deficiency) left in your body. Water is a critical part of health in your body, and dehydration can lead to kidney problems, migraines, spinal compression, and cardiovascular problems. I'll talk more about hydration in chapter 13.

If you eat too much of the wrong kinds of fats—such as hydrogenated (partially or fully) vegetable oils, fried foods, and foods such as chips, crackers, and the like—you'll likely carry too much fat on your body, potentially straining your muscles and putting extra pressure on your back. In addition, since the body requires a delicate balance of different kinds of fats to avoid inflammation, too much of these "bad" fats will tip the scales in favor of inflammation, pain, and illness—not to mention the other common problems that accompany obesity, such as heart disease and diabetes.

We can have too much of just about anything in any area of our lives. I've touched on diet, but what about the physical body? Too much running, cycling, or weightlifting—without cross-training with other types of exercise, sports, or activities—can lead to uneven muscle strength and flexibility (muscle imbalances).

Too much sitting at the computer can lead to shortened muscles in the backs of the legs, which creates pain. Too much stretching, without strength training, can lead to weak and flabby muscles that no longer support the body properly, poor posture, and eventual injury.

We can expand this concept to our mental lives. Too much stress can weaken the body's defenses and lead to sickness. Too much anxiety can lead to tension headaches and irritable bowels—even panic attacks. Too much self-judgment can lead to depression and low self-esteem, which decreases blood flow in the body and robs the tissues of adequate oxygen supply.

All these excesses throw the body and mind out of balance, tipping the scales toward pain and other kinds of disease.

Deficiency: Too Little of Something

When I talk about deficiency, I'm talking about too little of something. Like excesses, deficiencies can cause problems in your mind, body, and diet as well.

If you drink too little water, you run the risk of dehydration and toxic buildup in the body, as well as constipation and pain. Eat too little fruits and vegetables, and your body doesn't get enough of the vitamins and minerals it needs to stay healthy, fight off stress, and lower your risk of experiencing illness.

As with "too much," we can have "too little" of just about anything in any area of our lives. If we consider the physical body, the first deficiency that comes to mind is too little exercise. In America, we're suffering from an obesity epidemic. I talked about too much of the same kind of exercise a moment ago, but for many people, the problem is too little exercise. We're moving around a lot less than we used to and performing far fewer manual tasks, which is creating all kinds of aches and pains, to say nothing of the increase in such weight-related disorders as diabetes and heart disease.

If we consider our emotional lives, we can see how an insufficient amount of quiet time is a problem for many of us. We're bombarded by stimulation from all corners of our existence—televisions, cell phones, traffic noises, loud voices, radios, stereos, text messages, e-mails, and more. Rarely do we take the time to go to a quiet place and reflect. This constant stimulation leaves us anxious and unable to relax, reducing the amount of oxygen that reaches the muscles and creating blood circulation that's too slow.

These deficiencies create imbalances in the mind, body, and diet—again, setting us up to suffer because of some upcoming disorder or pain condition.

Stagnation: Something Is Moving Too Slow

You've probably noticed that some of the examples of deficiency are the opposites of the examples of excesses. This is because of the balance—or homeostasis—our bodies require for optimal health. When the natural flow of things stops moving the way it should, it's called a stagnation.

Stagnation can be caused by too much or too little of something in your life—or by both. Simply put, it's the slowdown of the body's natural processes—whether that means blood flow, muscular movement, tissue regeneration, digestion, hormone production, or anything else.

In a healthy body, the blood flows freely throughout the veins and arteries, supplying all organs and tissues with the oxygen and nutrients they need, while carrying waste away. However, if that blood flow is restricted somehow, say by a buildup of calcium or deposits in the arteries, it slows down and clogs up the system. As your blood flow slows, your organs don't get what they need, and the resulting stagnation can have harmful, lasting effects on your health.

Imagine one side of a two-lane highway. As long as those two lanes stay open, traffic flows freely (usually). However, during times of construction, for instance, one lane is often closed, which narrows the passageway and forces all the cars into the remaining lane. The flow slows down. Now, picture this with blood flow, digestion, or breathing. Suddenly, the stagnation is no longer an annoying traffic jam, but a life-shortening problem that can't be ignored.

There are many causes of stagnation. Too much anxiety, tension, and fear all restrict blood vessels, as evidenced by the feeling of "cold hands." Too much sitting for long periods of time, whether at the computer or on an airplane, restricts the blood flow in your legs, and can even result in a clot. Too much "bad fat" in your diet can slow down blood flow and leave you fatigued. Too much strain on a muscle can cause a muscle spasm, which can restrict blood flow. Too little activity, too little stress relief, too little water, and too little stretching to elongate the muscle fibers all can lead to low (slow) energy and poor circulation. And poor circulation can lead to muscle soreness, toxin buildup, pain, and illness.

Every aspect of the body, mind, and diet can be adversely affected by stagnation. Take a look at the following two charts, first presented by Dr. Wiley in his book, *Arthritis Reversed*. The first shows how the three causes of all pain and illness are likely the root of your condition, and how they affect it. The second shows how the symptoms you experience are also related to excesses, deficiencies, and stagnations.

THE THREE CAUSES OF ALL PAIN AND ILLNESS			
	Excess	Deficiency	Stagnation
Weight	Every 10 lbs over weight = 30 lbs extra compressive force on joints	Underweight = more nutrition needed to help repair and reverse arthritic damage	Remaining over or underweight pounds can worsen condition, prevent it from repairing and reversing
Diet	To much glucose, carbohydrates, inflammatory foods, diuretic beverages	Not enough water, thermogenic spices, anti-inflammatory foods, healthy fats and supplements	Unchanged diet = unchanged condition and contributes to worsening of symptoms
Exercise	Too vigorous, jumping and high impact = tough on joints	Sedentary, couch potato, unfit, atrophied muscles, loss of bone density	Buildup of lactic acid, muscle spasms, loss of flexibility
Sleep	Over 8 hours daily can lead to lethargy, over tiredness, weakness, malaise and depression	Less than 8 hours daily = insufficient repair, lower production of serotonin, cramps, achiness and stiffness	Sleeping too long in poor posture can increase pain

THE SYMPTOMS OF PAIN AND ILLNESS			
Emotions	Stress, anxiety, worry, obsessing over your condition can lead to depression and feeling that nothing can be done	Poor mental outlook can lead to unwillingness to help yourself, lack of dietary control, laziness, loss of enthusiasm	Lack of passion for life, desires, loss of interest in things, activities and what life has to offer
Range of Motion	Pain, inflammation caused by flaccid ligaments, too much space between joints	Inability to move freely, bend joints fully, stand or walk without pain	Extreme limited movement causing frozen hips, knees, shoulder, fingers
Pain and Inflammation	Reach for NSAIDs, muscle relaxers and invasive surgical procedures	Trigger points, muscle spasms, throbbing pain in fixed location	Doing nothing to help yourself, potential for endless suffering

A Dangerous Cycle

It's easy to understand how these three points—too much, too little, and too slow—can all interact with and feed off of each other. You can see how too much of one thing often prompts too little of something else—with the entire chain of too much and too little resulting in energy and blood flow that is too slow, creating pain and illness.

Suddenly it becomes clear why the more common approaches to treating pain and disease—those that focus strictly on the problem itself—don't address the underlying conditions. When you visit the doctor for migraine headaches, you don't have a deficiency of pharmaceutical chemicals. Yet you leave with a prescription for those chemicals.

With a little digging, your doctor—or better yet, you yourself—can explore the cause of your imbalance and find a cure. In other words, what do you

Make a List

One great exercise you can do to practice the Wellness Model of Health™ and create balance between your mind, body, and diet is to simply make a list. Take a piece of paper and draw three columns marked "excess," "deficiency," and "stagnation." Then start filling those columns with things that you think you're getting too much of, things you might not be getting enough of, and areas of your life where things are moving too slowly or not at all.

Think about the mental, physical, and diet aspects of health as you're filling the columns, and just start rattling things off. Remember, the little things do matter: they add up to big changes in your health. One thing will lead to another. Before you know it, you'll have a page full of things that you can start to work on balancing right away.

Just keep in mind that while this is a very powerful exercise, it's also a starting point. Several important health factors can't be seen on the surface. Throughout this book, I'll recommend different health screenings and tests that you can use to make your list more complete.

have too much of, what do you have too little of, or what is not moving freely enough that is causing your headaches?

It would be a mistake to assume that only one of these three causes is the root of any health condition. In fact, it is usually a combination of all three of them that make a simple problem become chronic and seemingly complex. The first "cause" of an issue could be singular (i.e., an excess), but when not approached with the Wellness Model of Health™ (i.e., restoring balance), it snowballs and becomes multi-faceted.

The way to alleviate your pain or illness is to consider it from this three-part perspective. If you can categorize where you are in excess, you can then make changes to decrease and balance these. If you are able to list areas of deficiency, you can then take steps to improve these. Where you find stagnations, you can look for ways to "move them along."

Returning the body to homeostasis can be difficult and challenging. Without the understanding of excess, deficiency, and stagnation and how those items work within the mind, body, and diet, it's difficult if not impossible to return yourself to overall health. You may have been polluting your body with toxins found in foods, beverages, and the air, and then aggravating all of this even further with stress, tension, poor sleep, and bad lifestyle choices for quite some time.

It's a dangerous and self-reinforcing cycle.

How to Get Out of the Pain and Disease Cycle

To get out of the pain and disease cycle, you need to return your body, mind, and diet to a state of homeostasis. That's not always an easy task. The problem didn't appear overnight, and it probably won't be cured overnight either. But that doesn't mean you can't cure it at all.

To help you understand how you can finally take your health into your own hands and start working toward true wellness, this book will look in more detail at the mind-body-diet areas of your life that are impacted by the "too much, too little, too slow" causes of pain and illness. I'll also cover some of the worst specific problems and diseases that arise from the excesses, deficiencies, and stagnations in your life.

It does not matter what condition you have been diagnosed with, or what pain you may be in. The topics and strategies in this book can work for any pain, and any illness. When you strike the right balance within and between your body, your mind, and your diet, you restore yourself to homeostasis, and you regain your health from the inside out.

The secret to overcoming pain and illness lies in understanding where that balance begins. And a lot of the time, it begins in our minds. In the next chapter, I'll walk you through the impact that your mind has on your overall wellness, and show you how to turn your thoughts into a powerhouse of health.

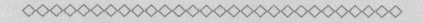

Chapter Review

- Mainstream Western medicine is based on a disease model of health; it treats the symptoms of illness rather than the causes of your condition.

- To achieve true wellness, three areas of health need to be addressed: body, mind, and diet. These are the foundation of the Complete Healing Formula™.

- All pain and disease is caused by one or more of the following three issues: excess, deficiency, and stagnation. Using these red flags to create balance in your mind, body, and diet is called the Wellness Model of Health™.

- An "excess" is defined as "too much of something."

- A "deficiency" is defined as "too little of something."

- A "stagnation" appears when the natural flow of processes in your body, mind, or diet stops moving the way it should.

- Excess, deficiency, and stagnation can become a dangerous cycle. To get out of this cycle, you need to return yourself to a state of balance, or homeostasis.

- No matter what condition you have, it can be improved or reversed by returning your body, mind, and diet to a state of homeostasis.

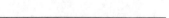

Recommended Resources

The Complete Healing Formula™

This two-CD set covers even more information about The Complete Healing Formula™: how the balance of mind, body, and diet impacts your overall health. To request a free copy, visit losethebackpain.com/chf-lpf.html.

CHAPTER 2:

The #1 Cause of Poor Health and Disease

Last Hope

I've spent a lot of time seeking answers to how healing can be found in the mind. One expert who knows a lot about this and who has a very powerful mental treatment plan is clinical psychologist Dr. Maggie Phillips, a friend of mine. She told me a story that demonstrates just how big a role the mind can play in the healing process.

Dr. Phillips once worked with a patient who had been through a series of terrible car accidents. Her patient, let's call her Laura, suffered from all kinds of pain: lower-back pain, sciatica, shoulder pain, neck pain. On top of that, she couldn't sleep. She had tried everything she could think of to relieve it. By the time she found Dr. Phillips, she had been through traditional physical therapy, ultrasounds, pain clinics, massage therapy, Reiki, and acupuncture.

"How did those approaches work for you?" Dr. Phillips asked her.

"Well, . . . " Laura admitted, "they all helped a little bit. But the pain still won't go away."

"What if I told you that you could heal your pain yourself?" said Dr. Phillips.

Laura was skeptical. She had been going from one specialist to another for a long time, looking for a magic bullet—one that didn't exist. She had very little confidence that she could heal her own pain. To her it sounded mysterious— like something she couldn't really learn how to do.

In that first meeting, she and Dr. Phillips talked about how Laura tended to let her mind get ahead of her body. Laura's self-talk ran along the lines of, "Oh, you should be doing so much better than you are," or "You know, it's really okay to sit in this position a little longer than you think you can." As a result, her body went into spasms, and she wasn't working productively on her own behalf.

Dr. Phillips helped Laura figure out how to put her mind and body back on the same page. Laura began practicing simple mind-body exercises. Within a few days, she was feeling better. Her confidence in herself grew. Soon she was sleeping through the night again.

Before long, Laura had achieved a much better quality of life and was no longer in the level of pain she had experienced previously. She had discovered the power of her mind as medicine, and it transformed her entire relationship with her health.

Mind Medicine

You know from chapter 1 that true long-term wellness has three cornerstones: mind, body, and diet. The cornerstone that Laura learned from Dr. Phillips was the "mind" piece of the Complete Healing Formula™, or what Dr. Phillips likes to call "mind medicine."

Mind medicine is a key part of finding healing. It's also the most overlooked solution to many problems. I define mind medicine as the way the mind works with the body in order to affect health. A lot of people refer to this as the "mind-body connection."

Mind medicine puts your mind and your body back on the same page. It gives you better sleep, better relaxation, and better confidence. It helps you understand where you are in your recovery process as you return to a natural state of homeostasis. Once you accept that and bring all of your energy to bear on the mind-body skill, there is no limit to what you can do for your health.

Try It to Believe It

We live in a society where the phrase "too good to be true" sometimes comes into play. So much hype is thrown at us that we don't always know whom to trust. Because of that, many people don't believe that mind medicine is possible. They don't believe that they can use their minds to control their bodies.

But very few people these days would disagree that the body and the mind are strongly connected. The body and the mind have a natural partnership. People have even reported using "hypnotic anesthesia"—hypnosis or mental relaxation—during major surgery. If that's not proof that our mind is an incredible tool, I don't know what is. All we need to do is figure out how to use it.

One of the biggest hurdles of mind medicine is getting yourself to accept the concept that you really can use your mind in conjunction with your body to heal yourself. This is a learnable skill. My clients realize quickly that mind medicine is a behavior they can understand and use. Better, it's simple, it's easy, and you can take it with you anywhere you go. And better still, it builds on itself. Once you get started, you see more and more success with every day you practice.

In this chapter, I'll show you how to conquer the biggest mental health hurdle we face: stress. I'll also dispel the old idea that your mind is on one track, your body is on the other, and the two will seldom meet. Finally, I'll walk you through the "pain gateway" and show you some simple exercises you can use right now to connect your body to your mind.

Stress: Is It All in Your Mind?

When you think of mental wellness, the first word that probably comes to mind is "stress."

All of us deal with stress in our daily lives, and we've heard—rightly—that stress takes a toll on our health. But many of us don't realize exactly how big that toll can be.

Stress starts as a mental issue, but it doesn't stay that way. Once it starts, it quickly turns into an emotional and physical syndrome. Negative thoughts and an inability to effectively deal with stress are the root of almost every illness we have. So it's no surprise that, when you quiet down your worry and anxiety, not only do you feel better mentally, you also see an improvement in your physical health.

Dealing with stress plays a key role in the success of the Complete Healing Formula™. In fact, the biggest roadblock for most people when it comes to relieving pain or eliminating disease is overcoming emotional hurdles, and stress is a huge part of that emotional landscape.

I have clients who are willing to do everything right physically. They'll radically change their diets, they'll do inversion therapy to decompress their spines, they'll do stretches and exercises to balance their muscles, but they won't deal with their emotions. So even though they feel some improvement, they rarely see complete relief. You have to be willing to engage with all areas of your health, and that includes your mind.

So what are the facts about stress? And how can you listen to your body's signals to help you turn stress on and off?

The "Off" Switch for Stress

How does stress cause pain? And how can you turn it off?

Let's start with some basic biological facts. Stress inhibits our body's internal system for pain control. This system is run by neurotransmitters that we call endorphins. When you're stressed, your endorphins can't work the way they're supposed to. In other words, stress lowers your immune system's ability to fight pain and illness.

Headache, anxiety, insomnia, and irritable bowel syndrome are all common physical symptoms associated with mental stress. However, that said, the negative effects of stress are also specific to the individual. Under stress, the weakest system in the body will be the first to break down. For one person, that might be the liver. For another, it could be the gallbladder or the heart. In every case, when mental stress strikes, you're not going to like the physical effects.

So where's the "off" switch?

We can turn mental stress on and off by listening to our body signals. The only problem is this: we've trained ourselves not to hear them. Over the years, we've conditioned ourselves to override our natural responses to our emotions.

A common example of this is crying. As children, when we were tired, scared, or angry, we cried. But as adults, a lot of us don't do that anymore—especially men. We hold back the fatigue, fear, or anger that wants to express itself. We keep it inside, and when we do that, we deactivate our body's natural signals and ratchet up our mental stress.

Our challenge is to learn how to mentally pay attention to the body signals we've been ignoring for years. When you're stressed, your body will send you signals saying, "Okay, I'm tired now. I need to slow down or turn off."

A lot of us don't want to hear that message. We're engrossed in what we're doing. Our egos kick in and we say, "No, I want to stay with this. I want to get it done. Just one more hour." This is the conflict between our minds and our bodies. We don't want to listen to our body's basic stress signals, so we override the body's command to the brain. Obviously, the results are going to be negative.

When your body sends you clear signals of fatigue, heed them. If you do, you can avoid overstressing yourself, and you can begin to bring your overall state of wellness back into balance.

Relax, Max

When we're stressed, our bodies hold on to tension. To release that tension and return ourselves to a state of balance, we need to learn how to relax.

A lot of us have forgotten how to relax. Here are a few tips you can use to train your mind to eliminate stress through relaxation.

- Relaxation Tip 1: *Breathe.* Breathing is the easiest and most convenient tool we have when it comes to teaching our bodies to relax. Slow down. Focus on your breath. Breathe deeply and feel the breath travel through your body. In many cases, stress-related pain will disappear just as a result of breathing alone.

- Relaxation Tip 2: *Music.* In some cases, listening to music can be a way to soothe your nerves and get your body to relax. Set some quiet time aside to listen to your favorite calming music. Music can be a quick and effective way to relax physically, and again, some people have found that this alone immediately relieves their physical pain.

- Relaxation Tip 3: *Train Your Brain.* Just as we taught ourselves to suppress our body signals, we can teach ourselves to acknowledge them again. This is done by "training your brain" through things like sound therapy and positive self-talk. Replace your negative self-talk with positive messages. Tell yourself "it's inevitable that I'm going to feel better." When you replace criticism with these kinds of thoughts and feelings, you encourage a natural state of relaxation and you empower yourself to bounce back from stress-related pain and illness.

Keep in mind that, just like you would with any new habits, it helps to take action to remind yourself to practice these techniques. To ensure your success, write these relaxation tips down on Post-It notes. Put them on your desk, in your car, on your bathroom mirror. Schedule time each day to breathe, listen to music, and train your brain. Then watch your stress slowly melt away.

Everyone has heard a story like this one: Someone is diagnosed with a fatal disease and told she has three months to live. She completely changes her life. She stops working the job she hated, gets out of her bad relationship, and goes traveling around the world. She does all the things she's always wanted to do, and then suddenly—miraculously—she's better. The stress is gone, and the pain and illness have left with it.

Stress is part of life. Everybody goes through ordeals that are painful psychologically, physically, and spiritually. But when you work to eliminate or release your stress, you free yourself from the shackles that are causing you pain, so that you can live a fuller, healthier life.

Stress plays a big role in our overall health and wellness. But it isn't the only thing that connects your mind to your body. Your mind can have an amazing impact on your ability to deal with pain. Next, let's look at that connection— the "pain gateway."

The "Pain Gateway"

"Mind medicine" can do more than treat your stress. It can also treat your pain. Understanding how pain works in the body is the first step on the path to effective mind medicine.

The pain mechanism in your body is known as "gate control theory," or the "pain gateway."

The pain gateway was discovered by researchers Ronald Melzack and Patrick Wall, who first published their findings in *Science Magazine* in 1965. You can think of the pain gateway as a component of your nervous system that turns pain on and off. There are nerve receptors along the periphery of your body, close to the surface of your skin. These nerve endings pick up signals from a variety of sources—such as pressure, burns, cuts, and even emotional pain—and relay them to the brain.

Say you touch something that is burning hot with your fingertip. That signal travels up your arm through the sensory nerves in your central nervous system until it reaches the brain. Then brain processes the signal and sends a message back down through your central nervous system and out to your fingertip, and you have the sensation of pain.

The catch in the system is that on the way to the brain, pain signals are relayed to part of your spinal cord. When the pain signal arrives at the spinal cord, it either gets a green light and is relayed on to the brain instantly, or it gets a red light and doesn't go anywhere. This is the pain gateway: it regulates which signals are sent to the brain and which ones are not, thereby controlling the pain you feel.

The pain gateway has been thoroughly researched, and all the experts in this field agree that Melzack and Wall are correct in their conclusions. If you learn to control your pain gateway, you learn to control your pain. But how do you give those pain signals a red light the natural way, without medications? How do you close the gates on pain so that you don't even register it as a problem?

This is where the mind comes into play.

Connect Your Mind and Body

There are a few very simple things you can do to build a bridge between your physical experience and your consciousness, motivation, awareness, and intention. Once that bridge is built, you have a powerful pathway for healing pain and living a balanced life of long-term wellness.

The following techniques, taught by Dr. Maggie Phillips, are basic tools you can use to help you start to harness the power of your mind-body connection. Try to practice them when you feel worried or when you're aware that your pain has increased. And remember, don't just do these exercises once. Repeat them over and over again. You are laying down new pathways in your brain that will bring your mind and body together. That takes practice!

Before You Start

First, make yourself comfortable. Clear away anything that might disrupt or distract you for the next ten to fifteen minutes. Unplug or turn off your phone. Put yourself in a place in your home or office where you can minimize the knocks at your door; you don't want people coming to find you. Also make sure you are in a safe place. Don't try to practice these exercises when you are driving.

Find a Comfortable Position

Put yourself in a comfortable position, either sitting or lying down. If you lie down, make sure that you are not lying down in such a way that you could easily drift off to sleep. Going back to the mind-body partnership, if your mind is asleep, you won't be able to gain the full benefits of these exercises.

You should feel that your body is supported. Some people need pillows to support certain parts of their bodies, such as their neck, shoulders, arms, back, or legs. Do everything you can to make yourself comfortable, and listen to the feedback you get from your body. It will tell you what you can do to make yourself just a little bit more comfortable than you are already.

Exercise 1: Conscious Breathing

Breathing is a fantastic way to start to experience the mind-body connection, and you can do it in under ten seconds. The idea is to follow the path that your breath takes through your body. Start by breathing in through your nose. Notice the flow of air, and pay attention to the way your muscles expand. As you exhale, again through your nose, notice how your muscles shift again in a different way.

Take a moment to really feel the experience of breathing in and breathing out. This is your own rhythm—the most basic rhythm of your life. When you inhale, you may feel a pleasant sensation of floating. An inhalation followed by an exhalation makes up one breath cycle.

Follow your breathing like this for three to four breath cycles. At the end of these, you will have effectively brought your mind and body together: your mind is noticing your body moving as you breathe in and out, and you should experience just a little bit more comfort with each breath cycle.

This breathing exercise is completely portable. It goes with you wherever you go. If you can make your breathing more intentional, you can reap a lot of benefits.

Exercise 2: Conscious Relaxation

The second simple mind-body exercise you can do is conscious relaxation. This is simply giving your body permission to relax from your head to your feet. Muscles, tissues, tendons, fascia, organs—everything works together, and everything is interconnected. The idea behind this exercise is to consciously relax them one by one.

Begin with three or four breath cycles, following your breath just as you did in the first exercise. Then, begin to relax your body, beginning with the top of your head. Be aware of any tension in your scalp. Then move down to your temples, your jaw, and your mouth. Really give each of those things full permission to release tension and relax.

As your head begins to feel a little more comfortable, you can move down to your neck and shoulders. Continue breathing as you give your neck and shoulders permission to relax, letting go of stress and tension.

Now you can begin to move down through your upper and mid-back. Give those muscles permission to let go. After that, come down the front of your body, giving the same permission to the muscles in your chest and around your collarbone. Spend some time on your stomach and abdomen, as well as the ribs on both sides of your body. Let those muscles become loose and pleasantly heavy. Remember to include your arms, hands, and fingers.

Then move your awareness down to your lower back, into the lumbar area. Each time you breathe, feel those muscles loosening up a little bit more. Next, move on to your upper legs, your thighs, and your pelvis. Then travel down farther toward your knees, your calf muscles, and your shins. Include your feet and your toes. All the while, think of your breath as a stream that is carrying relaxation throughout your body to where you need it.

As you practice this second mind-body exercise, you may start to receive signals from your body that let you know that you really are entering a state of true relaxation. Some people experience tingling; others feel a softening. You may feel light or pleasantly limp. Whatever that feeling is for you, acknowledge it. This will strengthen your mind-body connection.

Exercise 3: Tense and Release

The third simple technique you can practice to start building your mind-body connection is tense and release. This time, instead of just moving your awareness through your body, you're going to create tension in your body on purpose, and then let it go. For many people, this creates a deepening effect. However, if this increases your pain in any way, do not do it; simply go back to what you were practicing in the first two exercises.

Begin as you did with the first two exercises, with three or four conscious breathing cycles. Then, when you're ready, start creating tension in different parts of your body. Some people find it helpful to create a fist. Bring your tension, stress, pain, or discomfort into your fists, letting these sensations gather there. Make your fists as tight as you can. Then make them even tighter. Hold your breath for a moment, and then when the moment is right, let it all go as you exhale.

If the fists are not quite right for you, practice tensing a different part of your body. You can try this exercise with your legs, feet, or anywhere else you want.

Exercise Your Mind Medicine

Practice these exercises for whatever length of time feels comfortable for you, whether that means seconds or minutes. Then go back and do them again. Each time you practice them, you will increase the benefits.

Mind medicine like hypnosis and the techniques above can be incredibly powerful. In fact, they are so effective that you have to be careful not to ignore the potential underlying causes that may be causing your pain in the first place. Remember the Wellness Model of Health™, and keep an eye out for excesses, deficiencies, and stagnations even as you practice mind medicine.

These mind-body exercises work, and they work every time. Although they are simple and take very little effort, they are mobile and they are effective. All they require from you is a willingness to open up to the possibility that they can work, and then to give them a try. The more time you spend practicing them, the less pain you will have, and the closer you will be to a life of long-term wellness.

Want to learn more?

You can listen directly to Dr. Phillips as she shares more information about mind medicine online. All members of my *Live Pain Free* family have access to every interview I've done, and my conversations with her are some of the resources members appreciate most.

I've distilled much of what Dr. Phillips had to share here. But I can't condense an hour of conversation into a single chapter. To hear it all, along with other interviews I've done on subjects like hypnosis and guided relaxation, join my *Live Pain Free* family. You can get instant access by visiting: losethebackpain.com/membership.

Your Mind Is Your Medicine

Physical therapy teaches modalities like hot and cold packs, ultrasound, and electrical stimulation. All of these techniques are used to accomplish the same thing: getting rid of pain. When you learn to use your mind as your medicine, you tap into the Complete Healing Formula™, and you no longer need any of those things to achieve the same success rate that these homeostasis-seeking modalities offer.

Take the time to educate yourself about mind medicine. Be open-minded about trying something new and different, and really reaping the rewards of it for your health. We can create so much more with our conscious intention than any medication can give us.

Mind medicine puts the power of wellness back in your hands. And that's not the only tool you have at your disposal. In the next chapter, I'll show you how sleep can revitalize your health and take your overall wellness to the next level.

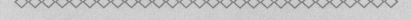

Chapter Review

- The body and mind are strongly connected and have a natural partnership.

- "Mind medicine" is the way the mind works with the body to control pain.

- Stress isn't just a mental issue; it's an emotional and physical syndrome.

- Stress inhibits the body's internal system for pain control and lowers your immune system's ability to fight pain and illness.

- You can turn stress on and off by listening to your body's signals.

- Pain in your body is controlled by the "pain gateway," a component of the nervous system that turns pain on and off. You can control this pain gateway with your mind.

- You can build a bridge between your mind and body using simple exercises like conscious breathing, conscious relaxation, and tense-and-release practices.

- Mind-body exercises can be simple, mobile, and effective.

Recommended Resources

Emotional Freedom Technique (EFT)

Gary Craig, the founder of EFT (also called "Tapping"), provides a comprehensive free tutorial of his tapping technique on his website. You can give EFT a try to reverse negative emotions. Learn more at www.emofree. com.

Live Pain Free Membership

Stay current on information related to stress and the other mental components of health and healing as a member of the *Live Pain Free* family. You'll gain access to more information from the experts discussed in this book, while also getting updates about the latest information and developments in health and wellness. You can learn more at www.losethebackpain.com/membership.

Dr. Maggie Phillips

Dr. Phillips has written several books on the emotional aspects of healing, hypnosis, and using the mind to aid healing. You can learn more at www. maggiephillipsphd.com.

Dr. Frank Lawlis

Dr. Lawlis is a prolific author, and has a wealth of information available if you want to learn more about a specific area of his focus. You can learn more at www.franklawlis.com.

Berceli Foundation

Founded by Dr. Berceli, the Berceli Foundation teaches his healing method of Tension and Trauma Release Exercises around the world. You can learn more at www.bercelifoundation.org.

CHAPTER 3:

Hidden Beneath the Surface

Look Deeper: Physical Pain, Emotional Origins

We are conditioned to believe that if we feel pain, something is wrong with our bodies. While that may be true, what we don't realize is that sometimes physical pain can have hidden, emotional origins.

Emotions are a natural and important part of life. However, according to Dr. Mark Wiley's book, *Arthritis Reversed,* in excess, emotions can be damaging to the body.

Here's one example. As I mentioned earlier, negative emotions lead to stress. Considering that we all have stress in our lives, it comes as no surprise that 66 percent of all signs and symptoms presented in doctors' offices in the US are stress-induced.

Let me repeat that. *A full 66 percent of visits to physicians who typically treat physical ailments are the result of emotional stress.* In fact, some estimates from the National Institutes of Health even claim that as much as 75 percent of doctor's office visits are related to stress in some form.

It doesn't have to be this way. Imagine what we could do for our health if we sought emotional cures for our emotional problems, rather than physical cures for bodily issues that are caused by our emotions. You know from chapter 2 that your mind and emotions play key roles in how you experience pain, as well as in the outcome of any program you undertake for pain relief.

It all comes back to excess, deficiency, and stagnation. Your emotions need the balance of the Wellness Model of Health™ just like your body and diet do, and your emotional balance affects those other two areas. Understanding this connection and getting on top of managing your emotions is a key component of finding relief and achieving a better quality of life.

This chapter will explore the connection between our mind and body in more depth, explain how we handle various destructive emotions, describe the vicious cycle of emotional distress, and detail the power that positive thinking can have on our bodies.

Follow the Signs: Your Mind-Body Connection

As you learned in chapter 2, there is an undeniable connection between your mind and your body. Our thoughts can actually create physical sensations.

Don't believe me? Close your eyes and imagine yourself stepping off a tall bridge. Your muscles tense up. You can feel your stomach fly up into your throat—all just from thinking about taking this action, without ever getting close to an actual bridge. A mere thought can trigger an entire chain of physical reactions, including dramatic fluctuations in your blood pressure, breathing rate, oxygen levels, and more.

Knowing this, you can begin to see the effect your mind can have on your body, particularly if you're in the habit of thinking stressful thoughts throughout your day. Your muscles tighten, causing problems like constricted blood flow—a stagnation. That stagnation can lead to oxygen deprivation in your body's cells—a deficiency. And that deficiency can in turn lead to the buildup of toxins and waste in certain parts of your body, which can then lead to painful knots and muscle spasms.

And the effects of negative emotions like stress on the body don't stop at muscle or joint pain. These stress-induced stagnations and deficiencies—not to mention excesses like cortisol, anxiety, and pain—are the direct cause of problems like migraines, high blood pressure, and other chronic ailments.

Another example of how the mind affects the body is how stress alters your breathing. Typically, when you're anxious or upset, your breath becomes shallow, reducing oxygen flow to your entire body. Stress can also release hormones, such as adrenaline, which can trigger chronic tension and inflammation in your muscles, ligaments, and tendons, leading to imbalance, and thus to pain and discomfort.

The bottom line is that stress erodes your health and undermines your quality of life. It is a psychosomatic response to what is happening around you.

In decades past, the term psychosomatic was primarily used by psychologists to identify pain or illnesses that were assumed to be "all in the mind" of the patient and, therefore, "not real." This outlook is dated and false. The seed of the physical condition is in the thoughts and emotions of the person affected by them. Indeed, they exist in very real forms, like inflammation, swelling, spasms, pain, and depression.

But how does mental and emotional stress begin to physically affect our bodies?

What happens when you are under stress—whether real or perceived—is that your body moves through a mechanism called a stress response. Through this physiological mechanism of stress, your muscles tighten, which inhibits circulation and restricts blood vessels, causing stiffness, inflammation, limited range of motion, and pain.

Other effects of negative emotions like stress include nail biting, anxiety, a racing mind, obsessive thoughts, compulsive behavior, unending worry, muscle tension and spasm, poor appetite, overeating, digestive disorders, constipation, insomnia, belabored breathing, neck pain, and shoulder tension, to name a few.

More than that, stress can cause us to adopt bad habits in an attempt to cope with the effects of our negative emotions. These bad habits can include dependence on alcohol, drugs, or painkillers, as well as the excessive consumption of food and caffeine. These misguided coping strategies then either cause or further complicate even greater negative effects on the body.

We have all the proof we need that what's happening in our mind manifests in our physical selves.

Take Control

Once you understand the power of the mind-body connection, you begin to see that our thoughts and emotions, and how we handle them, all have a profound effect on our everyday health and well-being. This means that during periods of excess stress, the mind-body connection can lead to new or worsening physical discomfort or injury.

It's unfortunate that as children we're rarely taught how to deal with our feelings. Generally, while we were learning all about reading, writing, math, and science, we learned very little about the art of mastering our own emotions.

If we were angry and blew up, most likely we were sent to our rooms, or if we were in school, to the principal's office. If we were depressed, many of us were told to snap out of it or to stop feeling sorry for ourselves.

As teens, we were more likely to get lectures and lose privileges than to have honest conversations about how we were feeling. However, those of us fortunate enough to have received some instruction along the way may have avoided the aches and pains that come from raging emotions.

Psychology has shown us that, by far, the most dangerous way to handle emotions is to deny or repress them. If we don't learn to express what we feel in a healthy way, those negative emotions stay in our bodies, sometimes for years, steadily wearing away our resistance to their destructive powers.

Learning to properly express and deal with our emotions is one of the best things we can do for our overall health, and especially for chronic pain.

Destructive Emotions

I talked about the damaging impact of stress in chapter 2. Now let's break it down even further. When we consider the effects emotions can have on our systems, we can imagine four different levels of severity.

Level 1: Everyday Stress

Level one is the everyday stress we're all subjected to, especially with today's fast-paced lifestyle. The morning commute, the demands of the job, watching over our children, managing our relationships, and dealing with daily crises like no milk, flat tires, forgotten lunches, scraped knees, visiting relatives, broken sinks, unpaid bills, and sick cats.

Most of us handle these types of stressors fairly well, but there's no doubt that unless we are consciously aware of the tension they can cause, they can still affect our bodies negatively. Without realizing they're doing it, many people "hold" tension in their shoulders by clenching those muscles, forgetting to "let go" of their stress by physically relaxing their bodies.

When these muscles are locked up for long periods of time, blood flow slows down and the unlocking mechanism stops working. The resulting trigger point or knot can be the beginning of muscle pain. If we don't take the time to unwind, burn off stress through exercise, or relax when the day is over, we may carry that tension to bed, where it will disrupt sleep and interrupt the healing process the body normally conducts at night.

The negative impact of prolonged stress goes well beyond slow blood flow and pain-causing tension. Numerous studies have shown a direct connection between prolonged, high stress levels and a decline in adrenal and thyroid function, which lie at the roots of several chronic ailments.

The bottom line is this: little stresses can pile up until the body reaches a tipping point, and that's when the serious problems start.

Level 2: Stressful Occurrences

In addition to the stress in our everyday lives, we can sometimes experience events that aren't necessarily out of the ordinary, but that ratchet up our stress levels nonetheless.

A car accident, even if we're not hurt, can rattle us and cause tension that lasts for hours. A promotion or demotion at work can create weeks of anxiety as we adapt to the new position. If one of our children is struggling in school, we may spend hours worrying, contacting teachers, and trying to set up help for the child.

Unexpected expenses, such as a house repair when we don't have the money for it, can elevate our stress levels. Strained relationships with our spouses or other relatives can stir our stomachs for months.

These events could all be considered "level two" stressors—those that aren't part of our normal day-to-day existence, but that can disrupt our regular routines. Again, how we deal with these events is more important than the events themselves. If we feel confident that we can handle them and take gradual steps to do so, we'll feel much better than if we feel victimized ("Why me?") or incapable of solving such problems.

Like level one stressors, level two stressors can constrict blood flow (so it moves "too slowly" through the body), creating trigger points or knots and, ultimately, pain and illness. The difference is that level two stressors can accelerate the process so that pain results much more quickly and/or becomes more severe.

Level 3: Major Life Events

As I mentioned earlier, we also have to deal with the "top five" stressors in life: death, job changes, marriage, divorce, and personal injury.

Experiencing any of these events puts a heavy load on your system. This is when you must call on all your resources for help: family and friends, support groups, counselors, doctors, massage therapists, personal trainers, and more.

No matter how you look at it, these events are going to affect you both physically and emotionally. The key is to put in place all the support you can so that you can recover as quickly as possible.

Maintaining a healthy diet, exercising regularly, and talking or journaling about your feelings all can help you cope.

One thing we often run up against in these situations is the resistance to taking care of ourselves. It's not that we're incapable of self-care, but that self-care has a negative connotation for us. It's difficult to admit that we need some time off, a vacation, someone to talk to, and someone to help us. Too often, we dive right back into our usual routines without taking the time to process and reflect on the situation that has just affected us so profoundly.

If you suffer a personal injury, such as a broken leg, severed limb, or heart attack, you're forced to remain in the hospital for a certain length of time. Your body requires that you be still and rest in order to properly recover. We accept this without question.

Yet, we're reluctant to believe that our minds and emotions need similar recovery time after, say, a death in the family or a divorce. This doesn't make any sense. Rest and recovery is necessary after any trauma—whether the trauma is physical or emotional in nature.

In these instances, taking time to get away for a while, to reflect, to journal, and to provide ourselves proper care goes a long way toward helping us avoid physical pain in the future.

Level 4: Buried Emotions—The Most Destructive Kind

At level four, we encounter the most destructive emotions of all: those that are repressed or buried.

Most often, these come about as a result of trauma, either in our childhood or adulthood, which we never completely understood or processed. Childhood abuse and abandonment, rape, and being witness to a murder or other violence are all examples of this type of trauma. Wartime events fall under this category; such incidents can haunt soldiers for years.

These experiences have huge, catastrophic effects on our minds and our bodies and, if not processed thoroughly, can lodge themselves inside us where they will continue to hurt us for years to come.

Repressed emotions, like anger, anxiety, and fear, can tighten muscles, reducing blood flow to areas such as the back and the neck—leading to pain and illness. Many times, this is an unconscious reaction to the old trauma, and the person is not even aware of the emotion causing the pain.

As I mentioned in chapter 1, in the 1970s, Dr. John Sarno, a professor at the New York University School of Medicine, first identified this emotionally caused form of pain, called Tension Myositis Syndrome (TMS). According to Dr. Sarno, TMS doesn't respond to normal pain treatments; instead, it keeps coming back because the underlying cause is untreated, repressed emotions.

The key to solving this type of pain is for the patient to become aware of the sometimes "hidden" emotions causing it. Dr. Sarno and other doctors advise patients to "think psychological."

For individuals who have gone through the usual tests and found no physical problems causing their pain, the technique of reflecting on one's emotional state can be especially helpful. In other words, when the pain strikes, instead of thinking about the part of the body that must be damaged ("Oh, there goes my herniated disc" or "Ouch, that muscle is getting me again"), the patient is told to understand that the body is perfectly fine and to think about what emotion could be at the root of the pain.

Taking the time to do some thinking about the emotions that might be causing your pain could be the key to your cure. Oftentimes, simply acknowledging the psychological aspect of the pain and identifying the problematic emotion can diminish its power within days.

The Vicious Cycle

Acknowledging the true source of your discomfort and poor health is crucial for your recovery. Even if pain and illness are caused by physical factors, emotions can delay recovery when we ignore them. For example, many people who suffer from pain caused by physical factors often feel very frustrated by the experience.

Frustration is an emotional stressor—which, as you may have guessed, can slow blood flow and make pre-existing pain and illness even worse. This then doubles the frustration level and the whole cycle repeats itself. Eventually, you may even start to feel helpless—like there's no hope for your health or your quality of life.

Negative emotions feed into pain and illness. This is another reason why it's so important to solve your health challenge as quickly as possible—so the pain or illness will not become chronic. If we try to go about "life as usual," we'll probably fail to give our bodies (and minds) the attention they need to heal properly, and then we'll be saddled with pain and disease for weeks, months, or even years.

This is a dangerous situation because it can be much harder to fix chronic pain and illness than it is to fix pain and sickness that has existed for only a short time. Once chronic pain and disease takes hold, it becomes much more difficult to fend off emotions like frustration and anxiety, which only make the problem hang around longer.

It doesn't help that so often our medical community suggests drugs or surgery for pain and illness symptoms. These "solutions" can cause people stress, anxiety, and fear, and when they don't cure the problem, they've actually made it worse by ratcheting up the anxiety surrounding the whole situation—not to mention all kinds of dangerous and sometimes even deadly side effects. We've been conditioned to believe that we are helpless and only someone else can heal us, instead of believing the truth: that we have the power to fight back within ourselves.

The effect of such prolonged or recurring stress is that is keeps the autonomic nervous system from balancing itself, which can lead to problems with the gastrointestinal tract, the digestive system, the respiratory system, and the neuroendocrine system.

The Power of Positivity

Just as your mind has the power to cause you physical pain and illness, it also has the power to offer you relief and true health.

A lot has been written lately about the Law of Attraction. The works of Abraham-Hicks, Wayne Dyer, Deepak Chopra, and Eckhart Tolle have given people a better understanding of the way in which our minds not only affect but also create our perceptions and our lives. If perception is reality, then what you think (the content of your mind) forms your belief system. Your belief system affects how you then see the world and how, in turn, you respond to it.

If you want to be healthy and happy instead of sick and in pain, you have to readjust your attitude toward health. Healthy people are happy people. And shifting your attitude from "nothing helps" to "I can make better choices" is often the key step that offers optimal wellness and emotional fulfillment.

Health and happiness represent a frame of mind that influences your choices. Making better lifestyle choices leads to wellness and a better quality of life.

It is therefore necessary—and actually, vital—that you work toward thinking positively about yourself, your life, and your condition. Let your emotions be your guide in self-regulating stress and its mind-body cycle.

When you feel bad, reframe your mind. Return to the Complete Healing Formula™ and pay attention to your excesses, deficiencies, and stagnations. Give yourself credit for the progress you've made so far. Looking for and finding the positive in all aspects of your life will attract more positive thoughts and feelings, ease your pain, and improve your health.

In the next two chapters, I'll take you to the opposite end of the emotional spectrum and show you how much power sleep and happiness can have over not just your mental health, but your physical health as well.

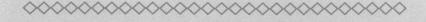

Chapter Review

- Although emotions are a natural part of life, in excess, they can be damaging to your body.

- The effects of negative emotions like stress include: nail biting, anxiety, a racing mind, obsessive thoughts, compulsive behavior, unending worry, muscle tension and spasm, poor appetite, overeating, digestive disorders, constipation, insomnia, poor blood flow, belabored breathing, neck pain, and shoulder tension, to name a few.

- The most dangerous way to handle emotions is to deny or repress them.

- The levels of destructive emotions include: everyday stress, stressful occurrences, major life events, and buried emotions.

- Acknowledging the true source of your emotional discomfort is crucial for your physical recovery back to optimal health.

- Just as a negative mind can cause pain and illness, a positive mind has the power to offer you relief and healing.

Recommended Resources

BrainSync

BrainSync is one of many companies that offers binaural beat audio programs. You can try their Deep Stress Relief audio program at www.brainsync.com/deep-stress-relief.html.

The Sedona Method Course

The Sedona Method is a program that aids you with improvement in all areas of life, including pain relief and recovery. You can find out more about it at www.sedona.com/Try-It-Today.asp.

Dr. John Sarno

As he was one of the first to connect the dots between the mental and physical aspects of back pain, I highly recommend John Sarno's books. You can learn more at www.healingbackpain.com.

CHAPTER 4:

Everything You Need to Know About Sleep, but Aren't Hearing

The Sensational Power of Sleep

Consider this: 71 percent of us don't get as much sleep as we should. The ideal number varies from person to person, but on average, most of us need seven and a half to eight hours of sleep each night. Even if you think you're sleeping enough, chances are you're overestimating how much you're getting. And some of us need more than we think.

Sometimes, the problem isn't about getting into bed; it's about what happens when we're there. Three-quarters of Americans experience insomnia at least three times a week. And the problem is growing. Nearly fifty-seven million prescriptions were written last year for people with sleep issues, a 56 percent increase in the last six years. The number of diagnosable sleep disorders has grown to eighty-nine, and there are more than two thousand sleep labs in the US alone.

The consequences of not getting enough sleep (deficiency) may be direr than you think. Sleep is a fundamental factor in the Wellness Model of Health™, and sleep deprivation increases your risk of hypertension, heart attacks, and stroke. It can worsen type 2 diabetes, and there are links between lack of sleep and certain cancers, periodontal disease, skin problems, and obesity. A lack of sleep throws your body, your mind, and even your diet out of balance.

It's obvious that there is a problem here, but luckily, there are also solutions. As a society, we need to stop treating sleep as a luxury and start viewing it as a necessity.

This chapter will discuss the different stages of sleep, touch on a few common sleep disorders, explore the consequences of sleep deprivation, and discuss ways to tell if you're sleep deprived. It will also help you figure out what's keeping you awake, offer tips to get your sleeping schedule on track, and help you determine when you should get professional help.

The Stages of Sleep: World Sleep Expert Explains

Dr. Jim Maas, one of the leading sleep experts in the world and author of *Sleep for Success,* says there are five brainwave stages in the architecture of a healthy night's sleep. The first two stages occur in what is known as "sleep onset." The third and fourth stages take place in what is referred to as "delta" sleep. Finally, the fifth and most commonly known stage is called "REM" sleep.

Stages 1 and 2: Sleep Onset

This first period of the sleep cycle, known as sleep onset, includes the first two stages of sleep.

The first stage of sleep is where the sleep cycle begins, and some argue that it's not even sleep yet. Here, the transition between wakefulness and sleep begins. The brain begins to slow down, producing "theta waves," or slow brain waves. Generally, sleep onset lasts around ten minutes, and when someone is awakened during this phase, the individual may not even believe that he or she was asleep.

In the second stage of sleep, the brain and body undergo more changes. As the mind continues to slow down, the body begins to produce more rapid and rhythmic brain waves. At this point, body temperature decreases and the heart rate typically decreases.

These two stages combined are what many people consider "falling asleep." They normally take place in the first fifteen to twenty minutes after you doze off.

Stages 3 and 4: Delta

The next two stages of sleep are also sometimes perceived as single stage, and they are characterized by the onset of delta waves. Delta waves are slow brain waves, which begin to emerge during stage three. The transition from stage three to stage four takes place when delta waves reach their peak.

At the Delta stage, the sleeping person stops responding to noises, activities, or other things in the environment. This is the stage when people are generally difficult to wake. At this point, your body and brain cells are restoring themselves.

Dr. Maas says that most of us stay in the delta stage of sleep for approximately one hour. Exceptions are senior citizens or people who take medication for things like rheumatoid arthritis, hypertension, or diabetes. These drugs, and others, often interfere with your sleep. Maas also notes that type A personalities generally don't get enough Delta sleep.

Dr. Maas says this cycle repeats itself every ninety minutes, driven by the individual's biological clock. It is important to note, however, that the stages do not always cycle through in order.

Stage 5: REM

Rapid eye movement, or REM sleep, is when 85 percent of dreams take place. This is the most well-known stage of sleep. The brain becomes more active at this point, making it the most likely culprit for the increase in dreaming and recalled dreams that people experience in this stage.

During REM sleep, voluntary muscles become essentially paralyzed, which forces them to relax. At the same time, several internal processes speed up. Respiration increases, as does the brain activity noted above. Eye movement likewise increases, which is where this stage of sleep gets its name.

For most people, stage 2 sleep precedes and follows stage 3 before progressing on to stage 4. The most critical thing is to have a full sleep cycle, including the restorative delta stages, before you wake up again.

Sleep Apnea

I've mentioned that there are many different sleep disorders. One of the most common of these is sleep apnea.

With a staggering 95 percent of cases going undiagnosed and more than eighteen million American sufferers, sleep apnea is a very dangerous disorder. In fact, Dr. Maas says that if you take sleeping pills or drink too much alcohol, you could literally die in your sleep.

We define sleep apnea as heavy snoring that causes repetitive pauses in breathing. This heavy snoring is caused by an obstruction in the airway passage. Sufferers hold their breath for thirty, sixty, even ninety seconds and then they gasp for air. This disruption of homeostasis can happen from six to seven hundred times a night, and you wake for a microsecond to resume breathing each time.

Those with sleep apnea find themselves exhausted during the day, but they don't know why. Those who live with someone who has sleep apnea can suffer because of the loud and continuous snoring that often the snorer isn't even aware of. The problem even goes beyond fatigue and lack of sleep, because sleep apnea can also lead to heart disease.

Danger comes in when alcohol and sleeping pills are involved because sufferers can be rendered unable to wake themselves up to breathe.

Weight also plays a factor in sleep apnea. Dr. Maas says that what happens is usually the affected person, typically (though not exclusively) an overweight male, has his upper airway obstructed. This causes the throat muscles to collapse, blocking the lungs from getting air until he wakes up.

One step toward relief is to lose weight. Another step is to outfit the sufferer with a CPAP, or a continuous positive airway pressure machine. A CPAP sends a steady stream of air pressure through the nasal cavity with a small mask that is worn through the night to keep the airway passage open.

If left untreated, the heavy breathing, gasping, and snoring can build up heart muscle around the left ventricle by squeezing it, reducing its size and increasing your blood pressure. This makes fatal heart attacks and strokes more likely, in addition to the everyday dangers of sleeplessness.

Because many are in denial about their sleep apnea, or they have apprehension about using a CPAP, they choose not to get treatment. If someone you care about doesn't want to get help for whatever reason, remind him or her that the treatment is crucial for their longevity and that it is noninvasive. Be sure to add that following treatment they will experience energy levels that they didn't know were possible.

Consequences of Sleep Deprivation

No matter what's causing your sleeplessness, the consequences of this serious deficiency are both numerous and dangerous. One danger is becoming drowsy at inappropriate times. In an interview I had with him, Dr. Maas cited the example of micro-sleeping while you're behind the wheel. You can fall asleep for thirty to sixty seconds with your eyes wide open; meanwhile, your brain is fully asleep.

I mentioned earlier that sleep deprivation can be a factor in hypertension, heart attacks, stroke, type 2 diabetes, some cancers, periodontal disease, skin problems, and obesity. But as bad as those are, the list doesn't stop there. There are also consequences to lack of sleep that don't manifest themselves physically. Losing your sense of humor, not wanting to socialize, and not liking to perform teamwork are all possible side effects of sleep deprivation that impact the quality of your daily life.

Dr. Maas says that basically anything that requires motor skills will suffer from sleep deprivation. For example, your golf game or piano playing will not be at your usual level.

Decreased cognitive performance is another risk. You may have a reduced ability to process material, concentrate, remember, communicate, write or speak well, multitask, and be creative when you haven't gotten enough sleep.

Your decision-making can also be affected by inadequate sleep, which can make for bad calls whether it concerns your stocks or your behind-the-wheel judgment.

Something else to consider is your workplace performance. This is a time when less does not equal more. Dr. Maas talks about a person up for hire or a promotion at work. When the boss asks the person how many hours of sleep they get each night, they might answer that they only need six, thinking that it makes them sound tough and efficient. In reality, if you hire someone who only sleeps six hours a night, you're hiring someone who potentially suffers from the above-mentioned consequences.

Dr. Maas, who is also a professor, says it's no coincidence that when he's giving final exams, everybody is coughing and sneezing. Long hours spent cramming and fewer hours spent asleep make students especially susceptible to sickness.

How to Tell If You're Sleep Deprived

Do you fall asleep as soon as your head hits the pillow? If you're on a flight, are your eyes closed before the cabin door shuts? Do you boast that you can sleep anytime, anywhere?

If so, Dr. Maas says you are pathologically sleep deprived. He likens it to having someone place a fifteen-course French meal in front of you. If you eat it in two minutes, it isn't good nutrition—it just means you are starving. So for those of you who fall asleep right away, you are starved for sleep.

There are five questions Dr. Maas asks to determine whether people are sleep deprived:

1. Do warm rooms, boring meetings, heavy meals, or lots of alcohol make you drowsy?
2. Are you asleep within five minutes of getting into bed?
3. Do you rely on an alarm clock to wake up?
4. Are you constantly hitting the snooze button on your alarm clock?
5. Do you sleep more on your days off?

According to Dr. Maas, if you answer yes to two or more of these questions, you may be pathologically sleep deprived and you should make a change in order to live a long, active, healthy, and energetic life. However, if you answered "yes" to two or more of the questions and feel that you *are* getting enough sleep, your hormones may be off; your adrenal glands may be fatigued and your cortisol levels may be high or low. Look into it, and figure out where you have an excess, deficiency, or stagnation in your health.

What's Keeping You Awake?

Sleep is often considered a luxury when, in actuality, it is anything but.

Maybe you think you only need six or six-and-a-half hours of sleep. Chances are, if you were to get that extra hour, you would say, "I never knew what it was like to be awake before." Rather than consider a full eight hours of sleep as indulgent, we need to view it as necessary and plan accordingly.

Kids typically need nine and a quarter hours of sleep in order to be fully alert the next day. Many kids are getting six hours, which is three less than they need. Homework, sports, social life, and stress about college are all contributing factors. But the biggest culprit by far, Dr. Maas says, is Facebook. He said that kids are spending four to five hours nightly online.

And it's not just kids. A recent survey said that 95 percent of Americans watch TV, play computer games, or are online within one hour of going to bed. There are many reasons why this is not good. One reason is that these activities can get your adrenaline going. But the worst thing is that our TVs, monitors, iPads and the like emit bright daylight spectrum blue light, which is an alerting mechanism. He likens it to going out into the bright daylight for an hour or two and then trying to go right to sleep.

Dr. Maas adds that the blue light is what drives our biological clock and our circadian rhythm. If you must use your devices close to bedtime, he suggests an app that cuts out the blue light or daylight spectrum blocking glasses.

In addition to the physical stimulants that disrupt our sleep patterns, society can play a part as well.

Some people have trouble saying no. They have a hard time reconciling that they have limitations and they end up compensating for this by sleeping less. But this compromises your health, and you have to realize that it isn't possible to go to school, then go to work, then go to practice, do homework, and expect to get a full night's sleep. Realistically, something has to give, but it shouldn't be your sleep.

I believe most people are spending way too much time on devices, and not nearly enough time resting. Resting includes sleep, and even goes beyond it: being alone, being out in nature, having time to think. Our go-go-go lifestyles are one of the biggest causes of disease.

If you have an addiction to technology, try to wean yourself off of it. Start by taking short periods of time to yourself. Even an hour will help. Then increase the amount of time until you can go days without cell phones, iPads, laptops,

TVs, and radios in your space. Just be alone with yourself, and you'll start to see the restorative effects of true rest.

How to Get Your Sleep Schedule on Track

Once you admit that you need a full night of rest, there are a few basic guidelines you can follow to ensure it.

Dr. Maas says that you should keep your room quiet and dark, and that you should set the temperature to be about sixty-seven degrees, though your best bet is to find the temperature that feels comfortable to you. Keep no clocks, TVs, or other devices nearby.

I personally recommend avoiding caffeine completely. We don't need it, and most people overuse it and burn out their adrenal glands in the process, forcing themselves to power through when their bodies are really asking to rest and recharge. But if you absolutely have to have that cup of coffee, stop your caffeine intake after two o'clock in the afternoon. Also, consider spacing out your coffee and drinking two ounces per hour rather than a single giant serving in the morning.

You should also avoid alcohol within three hours of bedtime, as it is a stimulant. While you may think that you slept great following drinking alcohol, Dr. Maas says that though you may have fallen right asleep, you were up every ninety minutes after that in REM sleep.

This next tip might come as a surprise: that early morning workout routine that has you up before the sun could be damaging you. Dr. Maas says that anyone who gets up early and exercises first thing is actually doing themselves harm. He cautions that it is dangerous to be running on a treadmill when what you should be doing is sleeping.

Even if you are getting your full eight hours of sleep, avoid the temptation to immediately begin pounding the pavement, unless that feels very natural to you. Try stretching for at least thirty minutes first, because overnight fluid builds between the discs in your spinal cord, and if you don't release the pressure prior to exercising, this can lead to lower back problems and possibly a herniated disc.

Plan your workouts for the time of day when you feel the most energized. Many people find that exercising between five and seven o'clock in the evening. or at lunchtime gives them optimal results.

A hot bath right before bed and some easy stretching will increase your body temperature, and then it will plummet when you get into bed, which will lull you into a deep sleep faster and for longer.

For type A personalities, set aside a "brain-dump time" to write down all of your concerns before you go to sleep so that they don't wake you in the night.

Dr. Maas also cautions against going to bed too early, which can induce inefficient sleep. You can try staying up late for a few nights and then slowly pulling back your bedtime by fifteen to twenty minutes a week until you're going to bed in time to get eight hours of sleep.

Ultimately, you need to determine what your own sleep need is and aim for that every night. You also need a regular sleep-wake schedule, meaning you go to bed and wake up at the same time every single day. Our body has one biological clock, not one for the work week and one for the weekend, and it's vital that you adjust yours for your optimum health.

Your Bed and Pillows

Many people ignore the importance of a good bed and a good pillow. I suggest a pillow that keeps your head, neck and spine in alignment as if you are standing up.

People tend to keep pillows for ten or more years, in which time they gather dust mites and begin to sag. One test to see if your pillow is good is to fold it in half, and if it doesn't spring forward, it's time for a new one.

Your mattress might also need replacing. It's been said that, typically, the weight of a mattress doubles over ten years because of the accumulation of dust mites. The next time you carry an old mattress, notice that it wasn't nearly as heavy as it is now back when you bought it. You can find my suggestions for great mattresses in the Recommended Resources at the end of this chapter.

Test Your Rest

Though you might feel you're being efficient by putting in an extra-long workday, Dr. Maas says anything you do after being awake for sixteen hours is worthless.

Try doing an experiment over two or three weeks in which you go to bed in time to get eight hours of sleep regardless of whether your work is finished. You will find that you are so much more efficient during your daytime hours that you'll actually have time left over at the end of your day.

Are Sleeping Pills an Option?

Many sleeping pills can induce a deep sleep, but with these, you won't get the ninety-minute cycle you need. Instead, you stay in Delta sleep (stages 3 and 4), and Dr. Maas says that is bad because stages 1 and 2 and REM sleep are crucial for memory consolidation and transferring the day's short-term memory information into permanent long-term memory.

This is where information connects with other concepts called mental memory traces, which boost performance. Your organs also can't heal and repair themselves if you skip out on your normal sleep cycle.

Dr. Maas says this is the origin of the expression "sleep on it." While you are asleep, your brain works hard to find a solution for any problems it couldn't solve during the day.

When to Get Help

I've covered several aspects of how your mind and emotions can have a positive or negative impact on your health. A rested mind is more able to deal with the stress of daily life or a painful, frightening medical situation. And more than that, it bridges the gap between mind and body, giving you a gateway into the Complete Healing Formula™.

Sleep is essential to the body's ability to heal itself. Earlier in this chapter, I discussed the link between sleep and heart disease, hypertension, and more. Many studies show that these ailments result from the inflammation that develops in the body from a deficiency of sleep.

If you have a sleep problem that persists for more than three weeks, Dr. Maas says you should visit an accredited sleep disorder center rather than your doctor. A primary care physician might offer you a sleeping pill, tell you it's part of life, or tell you to "suck it up."

This is why visiting an accredited sleep disorder center is so important. Even if your doctor is trained in sleep apnea, they might not be knowledgeable about the other eighty-eight sleep disorders known to exist. For instance, they might not know how to treat sleepwalking or sleep talking.

So when it comes to sleep issues, it's important to realize when to get help and where to get it. I recommend that you find a very experienced naturopathic doctor for this. You want someone who can look at everything that affects your sleep and your health as a whole, identifying excesses, deficiencies, and stagnations in your sleeping habits.

The right kind of sleep in the right amounts can seriously boost your health and quality of life. So if you're thinking that sleep isn't important or that you don't need it, you should put those thoughts to bed.

As important as sleep is, however, we can't stay in bed 24/7. The next chapter will demonstrate the connection between families and communities, and show you how you can use that connection to improve your health and wellness.

Chapter Review

- A full 71 percent of Americans don't get as much sleep as they should.

- Sleep deprivation can increase your chances of hypertension, heart attacks, and stroke. It can also worsen type 2 diabetes, and it may be connected to periodontal disease, skin problems, obesity, and certain cancers.

- The stages of sleep include sleep onset, delta, and REM sleep, all of which are important for restoring homeostasis in the body.

- Sleep apnea—heavy snoring caused by an obstruction in the airway passage—is one of the most common sleep disorders, and 95 percent of cases go undiagnosed.

- It's possible that you may be sleep deprived if you experience two or more of the following five symptoms:
    o Warm rooms, boring meetings, heavy meals, or lots of alcohol make you drowsy.
    o You are asleep within five minutes of getting into bed.
    o You rely on an alarm clock to wake you up.
    o You constantly hit the snooze button on your alarm clock.
    o You sleep more on your days off.

- Blue light from TVs, monitors, iPads, and similar devices stimulate our systems and interfere with sleep if used within one hour of going to bed.

- To improve your quality of sleep, keep your room quiet and dark, set the temperature to one that's comfortable for you, do not keep electronic devices nearby, stop drinking caffeine, avoid alcohol within three hours of bedtime, and don't go to bed too early.

Recommended Resources

Natural Sleep Kit

The Natural Sleep Kit offers a comprehensive natural approach to improving your sleep. You can learn more at www.losethebackpain.com/free-sleep.html.

Dr. Jim Maas

As one of the world's leading sleep experts, Dr. Maas's work has been crucial to our understanding of sleep. You can learn more at www.powerofsleep.com.

Recommended Mattresses

Looking for a mattress that supports great sleep? I personally use and recommend all-natural rubber and latex mattresses. You can learn more about great mattresses approved by the Healthy Back Institute at http://www.losethebackpain.com/back-pain-relief-products/mattresses.

CHAPTER 5:

Happiness: The Heart of Health

Heart-Healthy Happiness

Imagine this. You have two neighboring US towns. They're awfully similar—same mix of occupations and socio-economic statuses, same type of neighborhoods, same income level ranges, races, and even the same water and food supplies. But there's one big difference.

Town A suffers from the same staggering rates of heart disease and incidence of heart attacks as the rest of the county. And Town B is quite the opposite.

The residents of Town B enjoy unparalleled good heart health compared to just about everywhere else—even Town A, their nearest neighbors.

We've established that the people in these two towns eat the same foods, drink the same water, and work the same kinds of jobs. Many of them even work at the same places. So what's different for the residents of Town B that's keeping them heart healthy?

In a word: happiness.

Happiness is a powerful part of the mental aspect of true health, and we see that clearly in this example. The people in Town B enjoy strong family and cultural ties—so strong that no single person ever feels that they must face life's inevitable difficulties alone. There is always someone to turn to, someone to help them through hard times. As for the most immediate effect of this strongly woven community on its inhabitants, they are markedly happier than the average American.

What if I were to tell you that Town B was a real place? Believe it or not, this is true.

The real life Town B was Roseto, Pennsylvania, a charming but otherwise unremarkable village in the eastern part of the state. Two doctors in the area noticed this difference in the incidence of heart disease and coronary infarctions between Roseto and neighboring towns. On a quest for greater understanding, they teamed up with researchers to find out why—and just in time.

Before 1962, heart disease was rare in Roseto. The researchers started their work around the time that the US's heart health crisis was finally beginning to catch up with the people of Roseto. These investigators arrived in the town armed with the knowledge that this was a markedly healthier place to live, determined to root out the cause.

These investigators stayed in Roseto for many years, and their findings were published in the book, *The Power of Clan: The Influence of Human Relationships on Heart Disease,* by Stewart Wolf and John G. Bruhn. In this chapter, I'll share what these researchers learned about how being happier made the Rosetans healthier, and how we can apply the same principles to our own lives today to achieve the same results, using the Complete Healing Formula™.

What's Their Secret?

Since the 1960s, American consumers have been bombarded with information telling us one of the best and most important ways to avoid coronary heart disease is to reduce our intake of animal fats like butter, eggs, and lard.

So imagine our researchers' surprise when they found out that the normal diet of nearly half of all Rosetans, who had the lowest comparative rates of heart disease in the entire country, included frying much of their food in lard!

In fact, the time period during which the incidence of heart disease and heart attacks began to rise to meet the national average in Roseto came only after its residents began to change their diet in response to the national panic about the dangers of fat and cholesterol and their relationship to coronary disease.

That's right. After they started cutting out lard and eggs, the Rosetans started seeing higher rates of heart problems. This certainly flies in the face of the conventional wisdom.

Researchers have known for years that cholesterol concentration in the body is worse during marked periods of emotional stress. Indeed, multiple groups of researchers have found higher values of cholesterol during stressful periods than otherwise. But for some reasons, this understanding has failed to penetrate the national consciousness.

The Rosetan study revealed an even more important finding related to the Rosetans' diet and their hearth health. The Rosetans who were starting to develop heart disease consistently showed significant shifts in their eating patterns before the onset of the disease. And the number one related factor in the equation was stress.

During times of stress, Rosetans were found to eat much more or much less food than usual. A subsequent ten-year study of patients who had suffered documented, serious heart attacks showed a clear and highly predictive pattern of eating either more or less when anxious or depressed.

So what does all this mean?

Taken together, what these studies show is that patterns of stress are a better predictor of coronary heart disease than diet. Or put another way: happiness literally makes us healthier.

The Right Focus

Another major finding in the Rosetan study was the relationship between the happiness and health of the people to their attitudes about wealth and possessions.

Regardless of their income or educational levels, Rosetans showed a remarkable tendency to avoid displays of ostentation or flaunting money. In fact, this was considered a pretty serious taboo within their community, flying in the face of the burgeoning consumer culture that had taken hold of much of the rest of the country at that time.

Instead of shopping in the bigger stores in other, nearby towns, Rosetans preferred—almost exclusively—to patronize local small businesses. And when times were hard, the close-knit families and groups of extended family and friends in town knew they could rely on one another for mutually understood assistance offered in a friendly spirit of service.

In short, Rosetans looked out for one another—in both good times and bad. They treated each other with respect and knew they could count on one another. And while they lived this way, they were among the healthiest people in the country.

But as time wore on, outside cultural influences became more prominent in the town. Educational levels were on the rise, as were outside business contacts. Gradually, people in the town became less family-centered, and less willing to make economic sacrifices for the common good of the family or the broader community.

At first, Rosetans who enjoyed greater wealth than average were discrete in their enjoyment of this advantage. Weekend trips to places like Atlantic City for pleasure and entertainment were not uncommon, but when the vacationers returned home, their behavior was modest and circumspect.

In other words, wealth was fine, and having goals was fine too. But over time, the lure of consumer culture made its way into town.

People began to obsess over money, and they started working too much. A handful of luxury cars began to appear in driveways across Roseto. People who could afford to began to join country clubs. Short trips to Atlantic City were abandoned for longer vacations in Las Vegas and tropical cruises.

Soon, new estate-style houses began to spring up on the edges of town, far away from its tightly connected epicenter, where neighbors who'd known each other all their lives congregated in each other's kitchens and garages, keeping each other company from day to day. Life for families who moved outside of town was more luxurious to be sure, but it was also lonelier.

In the study, this loneliness (a deficiency) that accompanied the abandonment of the traditional, interconnected way of life of the town for a more modern, consumer-oriented lifestyle was shown to be connected to greater excesses of stress, anxiety, and depression, and higher incidence of heart disease and heart attacks.

Ruminating on the effect of this influx of materialism to the town during a visit to Roseto in 1974, reporter Robert Oppedisano wrote:

> What they gave up was the protective culture of peasant Italy . . .
> What they got in return was the chance to become Americans—
> rich ones, troubled ones, real ones . . . The past lingers in Roseto,

where rootedness and continuity are almost mythic qualities . . .
The present, for all its rewards—and Roseto is a prosperous
town—never fully satisfied" (IAM Magazine).

He got that last bit especially right. When we focus on materialistic desires,
we are never fully satisfied. But when we focus on people, the benefits to our
happiness and health are undeniable.

The Science of Community

One of the single biggest factors in the greater heart health once enjoyed
by the people of Roseto has been shown to be the extent to which each and
every person who lived there felt that they were an important part of a larger
community—a community that cared about them, that would always be
there to support them if and when they needed help.

Regular gatherings of community and local groups—combined with a
significantly higher number of three-generation families—made Roseto
a shining beacon of community support. Being part of a thriving, closely
connected community made the Rosetans happier, and thus, healthier.

Our understanding of how the brain works has evolved to the point that
new light can be shed on the direct health benefits of this kind of human
connection.

Here is what we've learned. Our brains process sensory input from the outside
world in a way that makes use of stored memory to interpret that sensory
information. While most of this process occurs, presumably, in the frontal
cortex of the brain, the behavioral decisions that result from this informational
processing are thought to open the electrochemical pathways known to act on
the heart, blood vessels, and other organs of the body.

In other words, our perceptions of our environment—and particularly of our
relationship to other people within that environment—not only strongly shape
how we think and behave, but also the messages that our brains send to our
bodies along the pathways of our nervous systems about how we feel physically.

The supportive social environment found in Roseto before the rise of
consumer culture there fostered a sense among its residents that they were
being nourished emotionally, which resulted in increased heart health. Over

the years, as this sense of community gradually deteriorated, the rate of heart disease steadily increased.

This goes to show how powerful the positive, restful social time we spend with friends and family can really be.

Happiness and the Mind-Body Connection

As discussed in chapter 2, it's well-documented that how we feel emotionally and spiritually has a direct correlation with our physical health.

The productivity of workers is known to be higher when they're shown that their superiors are concerned about their comfort and well-being. Similarly, babies who are cuddled and shown loving affection are known to be healthier than those who aren't.

So it should come as no surprise that when we feel lonely, isolated, or uncared for, rates of illness and disease skyrocket.

What this means, literally, is that paying attention to our relative happiness and connectedness to other people is as important to our health as getting enough sleep, exercise, and nutrients.

One place where this can especially be seen to be true is in the elderly population.

"Keep busy and stay active" is the common advice given to older people who want to stay healthy. This is of course in response to the phenomenon of elderly adults who see a rapid deterioration in health accompanied by higher rates of stress, anxiety, and depression after retirement and during the declining years—which are accompanied by the increasingly frequent deaths of friends, family and loved ones.

The stark truth is that when we cease to feel useful and wanted—or when we feel disconnected from our family, friends, and life purpose—our broken spirits result in quickly declining health, and all too often, accelerated death.

The Power of Gratitude

Renowned sociologist Georg Simmel once said that gratitude is "the moral memory of mankind." He went on to explain that if the sensation of gratitude and the actions we take in response to it were to suddenly disappear from human society, civilization itself would fall apart.

He is correct. Not only is gratitude the glue that holds our society together, but it may just be the ultimate key to living a happier, healthier life.

Social science research over the last decade has found that if we ignore the power of gratitude as a force for good in our lives, we do so at our own peril. Studies show that, unsurprisingly, gratitude is a key contributing factor to human health, happiness, and social connection.

One particular study, carried out by researchers at the University of Miami, sought to shed new light on the role that gratitude plays in human happiness. Three groups of participants were sought out for their first experiment: the first group would be encouraged to feel gratitude, the second, to be negative and irritable, and the third would be a neutral control group.

For ten weeks, all participants kept a short journal, with entries listing five things that had happened during each week. At the end of the ten weeks, participants who had been prompted to focus on what they were grateful for in these journal entries reported feeling 25 percent more optimistic about the future than participants in the other two conditions.

This in itself is astounding. But what's more, the gratitude group also reported experiencing fewer symptoms of physical illness than their counterparts in the other two groups.

In a follow-up study, a group of adults with neuromuscular disorders—including symptoms of fatigue, progressive muscle weakness, muscle and joint pain, and muscular atrophy—were put to a similar test. This time, participants in the gratitude group showed significantly more positive emotions and general contentment than the control group, and showed fewer negative emotions as well.

Also commonly reported: participants in the gratitude group felt more optimistic, and closer and more connected to other people. This was true even for many participants who lived alone and did not actually increase the amount of time they spent with other people.

What is truly remarkable about this study's results is that the change seen in the gratitude group was noticed not only by the participants themselves, but also by their loved ones. Reports the researchers received from the spouses of study participants showed that those in the gratitude group had begun to behave in a way demonstrating increased outward happiness compared to people in the control group.

Participants in the gratitude condition even reported sleeping more hours each night, falling asleep more quickly, and feeling better rested in the morning. Given that—as previously discussed—poor sleeping habits are one of the key predictors of poor overall health, this finding of the study gains added importance.

Cultivating a sense of gratitude in our lives is important not only because it makes us more likely to support and help others, but also because it has been proven to make us happier and healthier.

Live Happier and Healthier

In this chapter, we've seen that how happy you are directly affects your physical health, and that your happiness is strongly affected by important factors like how connected you feel to other people—particularly to your community and your loved ones—and how conscious you are of feeling grateful for the good in your life.

For this reason, tending to excesses, deficiencies, and stagnations in our emotional health and well-being is just as important to the Wellness Model of Health™ as caring for our physical needs. We need to take time to restore our minds, either through our positive relationships, quiet hours alone with ourselves, or both. Keep this firmly in mind as you continue along your personal path to improved health and holistic wellness through homeostasis.

I've taken you through several mental dimensions of how your mind can impact your health and well-being in the previous chapters. But as I noted in chapter 1, the Complete Healing Formula™ relies on three core principles: mind, body, and diet. In the next few chapters, I'll take you through the physical aspects of your health, starting with two key factors that most people overlook: toxins and parasites.

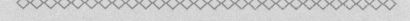

Chapter Review

- Patterns of stress are a better predictor of coronary heart disease than diet.

- When we focus on materialistic desires, we are never fully satisfied, but when we focus on people, we experience emotional and physical health benefits.

- Paying attention to our happiness is as important to our health as getting enough sleep, exercise, and nutrients.

- Gratitude is a major key to leading a happy, healthy life.

- Happiness makes us healthier!

Recommended Resources

The Power of Clan: The Influence of Human Relationships on Heart Disease by Stewart Wolf and John G. Bruhn

Learn more about the Rosetan community in this book.

CHAPTER 6:

Unexpected Invaders: Toxins and Parasites

Own Your Health

I am a big proponent of a fundamental wellness philosophy known as "self health." I believe, along with many pioneering clinicians and researchers, that you can take responsibility for your own health and well-being, rather than simply relying on others to maintain these things for you.

That's why a big part of the Wellness Model of Health™ is learning to understand your own excesses, deficiencies, and stagnations—so that you can correct them.

So many people are not used to taking care of their own health. Instead, they depend solely on the advice and treatment of outside sources such as doctors and other experts. And even though this paradigm is beginning to change, the misinformation out there sometimes comes with negative consequences.

For example, many individuals are beginning to taking control of their health through diet, though this sometimes leads to ill effects, given the various fad-diets currently on the market. Nonetheless, one big opportunity for everyone to practice "self health" lies in what we allow into our bodies—with or without food.

I am primarily talking about two things here: toxins and parasites. Toxins and parasites assault almost everyone on a daily and even an hourly basis, throwing off our natural state of homeostasis between body, mind, and diet.

Most people are aware that many of the modern conveniences we enjoy come with a price: exposure to toxic chemicals used in the manufacture of many products and articles we use every day.

However, less is commonly known about the extent to which we're exposed these toxic pollutants, their sources in our lives, and the specific health issues associated with them. Dr. Hulda Clark's work has been instrumental in shedding light on these topics, as I will explore in detail shortly.

But while most people understand that there are toxins in our environment, fewer of us are aware of the prevalence of parasites that also assault our health almost as regularly. Many are surprised to hear that there is a connection between parasites and illness. And yet clinical research exists that points to a connection between parasites like flatworms and illnesses as varied as diabetes, cancer, asthma, and multiple sclerosis.

This chapter will cover the dangers associated with exposure to toxins and invasive parasites, and how we can eliminate them from our bodies.

A Lesser-Known Cause of Infection, Illness, and Disease

Sick people want to get well. But historically speaking, in order to even have a hope of achieving this, they've had to rely on doctors, and on paying those doctors huge sums of money for treatment and medicines to get themselves well.

What if I told you that two of the leading causes of infection, illness, and disease were things you could diagnose and treat yourself, cheaply and relatively easily?

Dr. Clark's work on the root causes of all types of illnesses has yielded two ground-breaking discoveries. First, that the real cause of a number of illnesses can be traced to toxic pollutants and parasites. And second, that toxins can be avoided and parasites can be killed with electricity. In other words, if you're struggling to reclaim your health even after addressing the excess, deficiencies and stagnations you can identify, you should consider getting tested for parasites and toxins.

To be clear, killing parasites that have invaded your body and are making you sick will not make you well overnight. But it can jumpstart your body's natural ability to heal itself. Likewise, it can make the traditional medicines and treatments you receive from your doctors, pharmacists, and other medical experts far more effective—or even totally unnecessary—by eliminating the source of your health problems rather than just disguising your symptoms.

This life-changing information could revolutionize the way we understand and treat diseases and other illnesses. Imagine a world without diabetes, high blood pressure, cancer, migraines, lupus, and a host of other chronic illnesses that sap our health, energy, time, and resources, or even lead directly to the deaths of ourselves and our loved ones.

A world free of these diseases is possible if we educate ourselves about the effects of toxins and parasites on our health, and if we work to eliminate them from our lives and our bodies. Let's look at each of these two invaders one at a time, beginning with toxins.

Toxins and Your Health

It comes as no surprise that exposure to toxic chemicals and substances present in the world around us promote ill health.

Toxic pollutants are all the non-living things around us that don't belong in your body because they interfere with its ability to work the way it's supposed to. As long as they stay outside of your body, they don't pose a problem. This is why you can safely wear plastic eyeglasses and clothing. Unfortunately, these pollutants make it into our bodies far more often—and far more easily—than we'd like to imagine.

Our bodies react to invaders, large or small. You can probably recall a time when you had something stuck in your eye. Beyond just being an annoyance, your body increased tear production to try to flush out the invader. Eventually, the tears and your hands worked together to expel the foreign object.

Your body will do the same thing with toxins, whether the invasive toxic intruder is large or small, deadly or not. Like a militia defending its home turf against an invading force, your immune system will rush to do battle with this invader. Even at the microscopic level, this fact remains true.

In the form of environmental pollutants, toxins can invade your body through the air you breathe, the foods and beverages you consume, and the products you use on your hair and skin. These things come from places we're told are safe and non-toxic. And once the toxins are in your system, they start causing trouble for your health.

Types of Toxins

Many people are familiar with some of the basic sources of these kinds of toxins, such as commercial products used for cleaning, personal hygiene, and beauty. Likewise, most people are aware of things to look out for such as mercury in the water we drink and the fish we eat, heavy metals from old dental fillings, and fluoride in our water supply.

What is lesser known is that similar toxins are also present in our clothing, jewelry, and furniture. For instance, some types of clothing are treated with fire retardant chemicals. Some cookware is coated in chemicals that makes metal surfaces nonstick or scratch resistant. And certain mattresses—like any foam product—are manufactured using formaldehyde, a known carcinogen. Exposure to these things can make you sick.

The sad reality is that we are bombarded every day with toxic substances that can harm our health, and many people are unaware of the negative effect of this kind of exposure. Below is a list of the types of toxins we're exposed to every day, along with some of the effects they can have on our bodies.

Solvents

Solvents are compounds that work to dissolve other substances, and not all of them are unhealthy. In fact, water—which makes up a huge percentage of our bodies—is a solvent.

However, many solvents dissolve fats, which can make them very dangerous to our health. This is because fats form the membrane of every cell wall in our bodies, especially our nerve cells.

Solvents like benzene can enter our bodies through the air we breathe—especially if we're around a lot of cigarette smoke or gas fumes—and compromise the immune system. Other solvents that can harm our health include xylene, toluene, wood alcohol, methylene chloride, and trichloroethane (TCE).

Likewise, sodas can contain solvents such as methanol and isopropyl alcohol, which are known to attract parasites in the body. Commercially bottled water is usually packaged using plastics, which can allow chemicals that include solvents to leech into the liquids they contain. If you need to buy bottled water, look for companies that use glass or, at minimum, BPA-free plastic.

Even tap water is treated with numerous chemicals like fluoride. Spring water is the safest water you can drink, followed by well water, and even those should be filtered.

Metals

Our bodies need some metals to survive. For instance, the copper we get from consuming meat and vegetables is essential to our health. Inorganic copper, on the other hand—that finds its way into our bodies from water boiled in a copper-bottomed kettle or transported through the copper plumbing found in many older homes—is carcinogenic.

Mercury amalgam dental fillings, while deemed safe by the American Dental Association, should not be used due to safety issues. Even worse, sometimes the mercury used in this procedure is contaminated with thallium, which is even more toxic than mercury.

Pure metals present in the body spell trouble for our health.

Physical Toxins

Physical toxins are often breathed into the body in dust form. Our bodies typically react to breathing in dust by sneezing or coughing the dust out. You would never intentionally swallow a broken piece of glass, but if the insulation in your home or office building is left improperly sealed, that is exactly what you're doing—breathing in microscopic particles of fiberglass.

This means that any hole made in your ceiling or wall, however small, lets this in as well. Chronic exposure to fiberglass inhalation can lead to cyst formation—and cysts are a perfect place for parasites and bacteria to settle in the body and multiply. Fiberglass or asbestos—the latter of which has been mostly eliminated from construction materials at this point, but can still get onto your clothing via your clothes dryer's air belt—are often found in cancer patients with solid tumors.

Chemical Toxins

Some of the most common toxins in this category are the chlorofluorocarbons (CFCs) or Freon that enter our homes and workplaces via air conditioners and refrigerator coils. It's fairly well-known that CFCs are believed to have caused the ozone hole above the South Pole. What is less known is that cancer patients test positive for CFCs in their cancerous organs.

In her research into the link between toxins and poor health, Dr. Clark found preliminary evidence that CFCs attract other pollutants, such as fiberglass and metals, and encourage tumor-growth instead of allowing the body to naturally excrete these substances.

Other chemical toxins we're regularly exposed to include arsenic used in pesticides, and polychlorinated biphenyls (PCBs), which although banned from industrial use, are commonly found in most commercial soaps and detergents.

The bottom line is that if you're not really paying attention to your immediate environment or the things you're putting on and in your body, you can be exposed to a variety of toxic substances that can have a negative effect on your health.

How to Avoid Toxins

At this point, you might be a little shocked. You might even be thinking, "How can you live a civilized life if you can't use all these products?"

The good news is that, over the last twenty years, there has been an enormous growth in awareness about these kinds of issues. This has resulted in a variety of solutions to the problem of toxins in the products we use to make our lives better and easier.

This could be as easy as buying natural fabrics or pans made of a different metal. Or it could just mean using improved products for your household that are designed to be natural and non-toxic.

More and more companies are developing products that can get the job done without exposing you and your family to dangerous toxins. And with the rise of the internet and online product reviews, information about these products, as well as the products themselves, are available to just about anyone, anywhere.

Some people will balk at healthier alternative products and foods, complaining that they're too expensive. "I can't shop at the organic market. I can't afford that," they say. But meanwhile, they're watching TV, they're eating out all the time, and they've got cellphones. Essentially, they're investing in conveniences and entertainment, but they're not willing to invest in their own health.

Think of it this way. Sure, you can save money now by eating terrible foods, but you will pay the price for that decision later—even if "later" means decades from now. When you're seventy years old, do you want to be sick, hunched over, and barely alive? Or do you want to be strong, flexible, energetic, and healthy? That's what you're really buying when you invest in healthy foods and products.

It's true that it might take a little work on your part to do this kind of research and to hunt down these healthy products. Likewise, it's true that some of them are expensive, although this factor can often be circumvented using DIY versions that you can make at home yourself using inexpensive ingredients.

The bottom line is, if it means the difference between a safer and healthier home environment and lifestyle for yourself and your loved ones, isn't it worth a little extra work or even a little sacrifice on your part? What is better health—for you and for your family—worth to you?

The average American pays between $6,000 and $7,000 per year for healthcare. That's a lot of money, and it's sure to climb even higher as costs continue to skyrocket. Plus, as I discussed earlier, the current system isn't really health care; it's disease care.

Make an investment in your health by being more selective about which toxins you allow into your home and your body. You'll find that this particular investment yields far more return than a cell-phone contract or a new car lease.

Types of Parasites

The average person's understanding of what constitutes a "parasite" is somewhat misleading. Often, we tend to think of parasites only as larger creatures such as pests known to prey on our family pets, like worms, fleas, and ticks.

But smaller invaders like amoebae, bacteria, and viruses—whose presence on or in our bodies can powerfully impact our health—must also be considered.

We're used to the idea that we can be infected with a virus or bacteria, but we tend to forget that these are parasites—"things" living inside of us. Many people are shocked to learn what types of parasites (good and bad) live in or on us on a regular basis.

In short, everything living on or inside of us that takes its sustenance from our bodies can be considered an invading parasite—regardless of its size.

The most common larger parasites found in the human body, whose presence is known to be associated with diseases as serious as cancer and AIDS/HIV, are parasitic worms. As Dr. Clark's research shows, parasites in this category are divided into roundworms and flatworms.

Don't let the word "worm" give you the impression that these creatures are large and easy to spot. They're actually difficult to locate with traditional methods, but the damage they wreak on our health is easy to see.

Of roundworms and flatworms, flatworms are the most dangerous. Functioning much like leeches, these parasites (also sometimes called flukes) physically attach themselves in some way to their host, sometimes with tiny, sucker-like appendages.

Parasites and Your Health

What is still not commonly understood by the medical establishment or the general public, but has been shown in the work of researchers like Dr. Clark, is that the presence of larger parasites like flatworms in the human body often serves to pave the way for smaller parasites like bacteria and viruses to cause infection and illness.

Bacteria and viruses can wreck your health in and of themselves, and they typically bring other "companion" viruses and bacteria with them. These companions are what most traditional medical practitioners identify as the cause of an ailment. But in fact, the companion bacteria are simply the symptom of the true cause: the presence of the parasite.

What this means, in essence, is that if, unbeknownst to us, our bodies are harboring these larger types of parasites, then we are far more likely to contract illnesses and diseases than we otherwise would be.

How to Kill Parasites Naturally

Remember, parasites and their pathogens are living things and, much like us, overexposure to electrical current can kill them. Because of that, many parasites and pathogens can be eliminated using a small amount of electricity (as little as 5 volts). This can be done by "zapping" your body with a commercial frequency generator, a device that not only kills parasites, but will allow you to identify if they are present in your body in the first place, and if so, what kind or parasites you're dealing with.

Dr. Clark's book, *The Cure for All Diseases*, gives specific instructions for how to go about identifying and eliminating parasites through electrical zapping. The good news is that these electrical zappers described by Clark are not harmful to you. In fact, they are barely noticeable. But the impact on the offending parasites and parasite companions in your body is deadly.

Be advised that it takes three treatments of electricity to kill most small parasites. The reason for this is that the first zapping kills smaller parasites like viruses and bacteria. But only a few minutes later, other bacteria and viruses that were being suppressed by the dominant ones that have now been killed will be released and seek to gain a foothold in your body.

The second zapping kills the newly released bacteria and viruses, and starts this cycle one more time. But by the third round of zapping, the cycle is stopped—at this point, the harmful viruses and bacteria that you identified as being present in your body will have been eliminated.

To kill flatworms, roundworms, protozoa, and even bacteria and viruses, a combination of zapping and herbal therapy is recommended, using black walnut hull tincture, wormwood, and cloves. For specific dosages and recommended sources for top quality herbal products, again, see Dr. Clark's book.

Live Toxin and Parasite Free

As Dr. Clark's work shows, avoiding toxins and eliminating parasites from our bodies can have an enormous positive impact on our health—even helping our bodies rid themselves of serious diseases like diabetes, cancer, HIV/AIDS, and lupus. But it's up to each of us to educate ourselves about the dangers associated with toxins and parasites and how to rid our bodies of them, and to take action to make this happen.

While medical expertise is certainly important, and I am not advocating that you stop going to or listening to your doctor, it is equally as important to take ownership of your health by paying attention to and listening to your own body, engaging with the Complete Healing Formula™, and advocating for your own care.

It's your body, and your health. The only expert on the experience of the excesses, deficiencies, and stagnations going on in your body is you. Embrace a philosophy of self-health, and use it to eliminate toxins and parasites from your daily life.

Then, take it a step further. While toxins and parasites play an immense role in our health, they are far from the only physical factor we need to take into consideration. The next item on the Wellness Model of Health™ checklist is muscle imbalance, learning about which can very well revolutionize the way you approach your health.

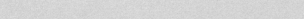

Chapter Review

- Toxins and parasites assault almost everyone on a daily basis.

- A number of illnesses can be traced to toxic pollutants and parasites in our environments.

- Toxins can invade your body through your air, water, food, and personal products—even when these things are said to be safe and non-toxic.

- Some common sources of toxins include: solvents, metals, physical toxins, and chemical toxins.

- You can avoid many toxins by making simple changes in what you buy and what you eat.

- The most common parasites found in the human body are parasitic worms. Of them, flatworms are the most dangerous.

- You can kill parasites and pathogens yourself using a commercial frequency generator.

Recommended Resources

ElectroCleanse

This tool, developed with the Dr. Clark Research Association, is crucial to harnessing the healing of many major medical disorders. You can find out more about it at www.losethebackpain.com/productreviews/electrocleanse. html.

Dr. Clark Research Association

You can learn more about the available tools that you can use to clear toxins from your system from the Dr. Clark Research Association at www.drclark. com.

Clark Therapy by Ignacio Chamorro Balda

You can also find more information about Dr. Clark's tools and methods in this book.

CHAPTER 7:

Muscle Imbalances: The #1 Physical Cause of Pain

Living with Muscle and Joint Pain

As humans, we can suffer from many different ailments, caused by any number of things. One of the top causes of suffering among American adults is muscle and joint pain.

Literally millions of people suffer from chronic muscle and joint pain, which can last for years, growing worse over time. In fact, according to researchers from the American Chiropractic Association, over thirty-one million Americans are experiencing back pain symptoms this very minute. What's more, researchers from the Mayo Clinic estimate that a whopping 80 percent of the population will experience back problems at some point in their lives.

Pinpointing the source of this kind of pain can be difficult, and all too often, finding actual, working solutions for ridding ourselves of this pain is even harder to do. If you're like most folks, you've probably been told by your health care practitioner that overuse of your muscles, poor posture, and even your genetic history are the primary causes of your muscle and joint pain.

Unfortunately, most doctors are dead wrong about this, because they are unfamiliar with the excess, deficiency, and stagnation framework of the Wellness Model of Health™. Health experts and back care specialists have found that the real, underlying cause of your problems is actually not your posture, the amount you exercise, or your genetic history at all.

The real reason you have pain is because your body and spine have been pulled out of their normal positions and into what are called physical dysfunctions. In other words, you're experiencing a lack of homeostasis. Physical dysfunctions are abnormalities in how your body operates. And they're caused by imbalances between various muscle groups—called "muscle imbalances."

If you have joint or muscle pain, there is an 80 percent or greater chance that muscle imbalances are one of its primary causes. These muscle imbalances are the hidden cause of nearly every case of pain experienced by the majority of people who suffer from back problems and other ailments. You don't need to go to the doctor to fix them. In fact, this is a great area to practice "self health."

In this chapter, I'll examine what muscle imbalances are, what they do to our bodies, what causes them, and how to fix them by paying attention to excess, deficiency, and stagnation in your muscular network.

Why Traditional Muscle and Joint Pain Treatments Fail

When it comes to pain, knowledge is power. It's important to learn all you can about your particular condition because informed people get better care and faster results.

A basic fact about pain is that most treatments fail because they begin at the end— that is, they merely focus on the pain, which is just a symptom of a larger problem. They don't look at your excesses, deficiencies, or stagnations.

A word of caution: if you feel even minor pain, you should take it very seriously. Your body is telling you that something is not right. Failing to address this situation now will likely result in a higher level of pain and having to work much harder and much longer to get yourself back to a pain-free state.

Whether your goal is to stay healthy or to get lasting relief from your pain, you should know that pain—or any disease, for that matter—develops as a process. Muscle Balance Therapy™, which I will cover later, addresses the underlying cause of your condition while at the same time bringing relief from your symptoms.

In essence, it attempts to reverse the process that brought you pain and bring your body back to a more neutral state.

The Greeks understood these principles as far back as two thousand five hundred years ago, but somehow this simple, sensible approach was replaced by today's medical treatments that merely focus on symptoms rather than the source of your pain.

What Is a Muscle Imbalance?

Chances are, you have never heard of muscle imbalances, and worse, you don't even know that your own muscles are out of balance. But the reality is that everyone has muscle imbalances to some degree—regardless of age, sex, or level of fitness. No one is perfect. And even if you did manage to achieve perfection, you could not stay there for long.

In simple terms, a muscle imbalance occurs when you have overdeveloped and tight muscles in one area of your body while the opposing muscles are weak and stretched out of their normal position. These imbalances can happen anywhere on the body and often develop as the result of the routine things you do while on the job, playing sports, or engaging in other activities you enjoy.

IT band syndrome, SI joint syndrome, sciatica, frozen shoulder, knee pain, hip pain, and all forms of back pain are just a few conditions that can develop as a result of muscle imbalances.

Why People Have Muscle and Joint Pain

As your muscles get more and more out of balance, you end up pulling yourself out of proper alignment, thus producing even more stress and causing additional wear and tear on muscles, ligaments, joints, and even the spine. This deficiency of alignment and excess of wear and tear results in a lack of homeostasis in your body and mind, which means they can't function the way they should.

Almost all of us live our lives with chronic unrecognized muscular imbalances. And while it does take time for muscle imbalances to cause a symptomatic condition, the first signs of trouble are evident in our bodies in the form of "postural dysfunctions." Postural dysfunction can be seen in the abnormal position on the pelvis, head, neck, shoulder, knee, and even in the curvature of the spine.

Once a postural dysfunction has developed, your body cannot go on for long this way before you will begin to experience problems. That is why you should never just cover up the pain or put off addressing your condition. In other words, if you are in your forties, don't wait until you're in your sixties to decide you have a problem.

Try this analogy. If you drive your car with the wheels out of alignment, the tread on your tires is going to wear unevenly. If you don't get an alignment, eventually you're going to have a blowout. The same principle holds true for your back and other areas of your body.

What is Muscle Balance Therapy™?

Muscle Balance Therapy™ is an innovative approach to eliminating most forms of musculoskeletal pain, and most notably, back pain, once and for all. It starts with a careful yet simple assessment of all the muscles that affect the stability of your hips, pelvis, and spine—from the perspective of both strength and flexibility.

Before getting started on any stretching or exercise meant to alleviate these muscle imbalances, it is critical to understand where those imbalances lie. The good news is that muscle imbalances can be diagnosed simply and easily by you in your own home.

It's important to note that, in the absence of these assessments, any exercise you might try is going to put you at risk of strengthening a muscle that does not need to be strengthened, which can make your condition worse. The same is true for stretching – if you stretch a muscle that does not need to be stretched, you could be doing more harm than good.

Once your assessments are done, you will have proved to yourself that you do have muscle imbalances and that you have one or more postural dysfunctions. You also will have learned the root cause of your condition. Best of all, you will know exactly how to correct the problem using the Complete Healing Formula™.

How to Use Muscle Balance Therapy™ to Finally Get Lasting Relief

Properly diagnosing your muscle imbalances requires a step-by-step process that is known only to a small number of health care practitioners. Unfortunately, it's difficult to find out which practitioners understand the principles behind this method.

You've probably heard your doctor, chiropractor, or other health care professional tell you to stretch or strengthen some part of the body. Perhaps he or she even diagnosed you with a condition like scoliosis or a raised hip/shortened leg, then gave you some stretches or a heal lift.

Stretches work—if you're stretching the right part of your body. However, you probably received a pre-made sheet of stretches with all or most of them "checked" for you to go home and do yourself. But have you ever wondered how the same stretches can work for everyone, regardless of the cause of their pain?

If you haven't, then this is the time to ask. The answer is simple: they can't!

Rather than relying on pre-set stretches and a "one-size-fits-all" approach, The Healthy Back Institute has created a program to allow you to understand where you need flexibility and where you need strength. It all starts with understanding your own situation—the same "self health" approach I discussed earlier.

Here is what you need to know about this Muscle Balance Therapy self-treatment kit that I developed years ago. This kit includes a video training program that shows you how your body should be moving when it's well-balanced. It includes reference photographs of how every major part of your body should look when sitting, standing, and walking.

This allows you to compare your muscle-balance levels to those displayed on the videos and in the photographs—making it easy to isolate what's causing your back pain.

Several videos show you exactly what the different postural dysfunctions look like in action. Unfortunately, video material can't be conveyed very easily in the written format of a book. Once you see the various dysfunctions and compare them to how your body stands, sits, and walks, you'll be able to accurately assess your own condition.

The other critical thing that the videos show you is the proper way to implement the corrective stretches and exercises. This allows you to see what an imbalanced body looks like, how to fix it, and what your body should look like after you're done.

The key here is simple: if you understand what postural imbalances you have, then you can understand how to correct them. I myself was diagnosed with scoliosis, but with no surgery, no doctor visits, and no expense, I'm "cured."

It is only rare cases where a misalignment of the spine (or any body part) is a true skeletal abnormality. Far more commonly, we discover that our muscles are pulling our skeletons in directions that they don't want to go. Fix that, and you've fixed the cause of the problem.

This same muscle balance therapy applies to any joint pain you have, from your toes to your fingers to your skull. Plus, strength imbalances in the legs and arms are usually a contributing factor in arthritis, tendonitis, and more. Again, the message here is simple: understand your anatomy, observe where it is not balanced (excess strength, deficient flexibility, or stagnant motion), and you can improve and heal these problems.

Take Your Situation Seriously

Once you've determined your muscle imbalances and started the targeted exercises to address them, you'll start to feel better quickly. Within days, you'll probably notice some relief, and if you continue the corrective exercises, you'll find your body making steady progress and your pain fading as you return to a natural state of homeostasis.

Free Yourself from Muscular, Skeletal, and Nerve Pain

Returning homeostasis to your postures, as well as your muscle strength and flexibility, will help with movement and reduce pain levels throughout your body. When you address the real cause of your pain according to your excesses, deficiencies, and stagnations, you can experience a cascade of healing through the Wellness Model of Health™.

A life free of muscle and joint pain means different things for different sufferers of this kind of pain. It could mean getting a full night's rest without waking up sore, or being able to work in the garden, clean the house, wash the car, or lift your grandkids without hurting for days afterwards.

You can start curing yourself of muscle and joint pain today. The Healthy Back Institute's Lose the Back Pain® System™ has been used by more than seventy thousand people in more than one hundred and twenty countries. You can learn more about this proven system by visiting www.losethebackpain.com/products.

I'll go into far more detail with some of the common conditions caused in part by muscle and joint pain in later chapters. It may sound too good to be true, but if you educate yourself about the real causes of your pain and try these proven therapies, you—like so many other people before you—will be astounded by the results.

Muscle imbalances are one of the biggest causes of pain. However, there's another little-known cause of pain that plays a big part in your physical health as well: trigger points. In the next chapter, I'll introduce you to what trigger points are, how they develop, and why they cause pain.

Chapter Review

- Muscle and back pain are one of the top causes of suffering among American adults. Approximately 80 percent of the population will experience back problems at some point in their lives.

- Muscle imbalances are imbalances between the various muscle groups in your body, and are the hidden cause of nearly every case of pain.

- Everyone has muscle imbalances to some degree, regardless of age, sex, or level of fitness.

- Muscle Balance Therapy™ assesses all the muscles that affect your overall stability from a strength and flexibility perspective so that you can work toward homeostasis.

- When you begin to address muscle imbalances, you can start to feel pain relief within days.

Recommended Resources

Lose the Back Pain® System™

I developed a system you can use to get rid of your back pain for good. The Lose the Back Pain® System™ gives you the tools you need to assess the real cause of your pain, along with simple steps to treat and cure the pain yourself. You can find out more at www.losethebackpain.com/getstarted.

Lose the Neck Pain® System™

Developed after the monumental success of the Lose the Back Pain® System™, here you'll find the treatment and relief you need for your persistent neck and shoulder pain. Learn more at www.losetheneckpain.com.

CHAPTER 8:

Trigger Points: The "Mystery Cause" of Muscle and Joint Pain

Behind the Scenes of Muscle Health

In recent years, the medical community has learned more about how our anatomy is really put together, and more and more fingers keep pointing in the direction of trigger points.

It's long been understood that our muscles are composed of tiny, microscopic fibers. These fibers connect to one another and to the body, allowing for movement and motion. What has only more recently been accepted by the slow-to-move medical community is that muscles are covered in something called the fascia—thin, fibrous tissue that connects the entire body structure from head to toe.

The fascia and muscles work together to allow us to move our limbs and feel various sensations. Truly understanding how this relates to pain begins with exploring the muscle fibers, which are then directly connected all along their structure to the fascia.

In a healthy muscle, all the fibers are long and even, like dry spaghetti, or like the hairs on the bow of a violin. They flow smoothly when you move them, just like spaghetti strands when they slide out of the package.

What Is a Trigger Point?

A trigger point is essentially a small, painful, hard knot within a muscle, which many people refer to as a muscle "knot" or "cramp." Trigger points are commonly known to be a cause of neck or shoulder pain, but they are less-commonly known for the role they play in fibromyalgia and other chronic pain disorders.

A trigger point causes an unhealthy contraction, so that some of those muscle fibers twist or seize up into a knot. Imagine a crooked piece of dry spaghetti, or a snag in the package: some pieces move and some do not. When we apply that image to a muscle, the implications are pretty clear. Some muscles move and others do not, leading to a trigger point or knot, and that causes pain.

When a knot appears in a muscle, it causes pain for two reasons. First, the muscle loses access to the nutrients in the blood, and second, without healthy circulation passing through, toxins tend to build up in the contracted area. The usual result of these problems is inflammation as the body tries to quarantine and heal itself.

Not only does this affect the muscle itself, but it also impacts other parts of the body that fall along the pathway of the muscle and the fascia. So although pain can manifest in the trigger point itself, you feel it even more often in places that are connected to it in the muscles or fascia.

In addition to twisting fibers, the muscle typically shortens as well, just like a strand of rope shortens when you tie a few knots in the middle of it. Because the muscle can't move as freely as it should, the rest of the muscle and surrounding fascia put extra strain on the area. This deficiency of movement and excess strain often restricts the range of motion and flexibility in the affected area.

The good news is that these trigger points aren't hidden or undetectable. Anyone can feel a trigger point. In fact, you've probably felt many on yourself or someone else many times. If you massage another person, when your fingers run over hard knots under the skin, those knots are usually trigger points. Or if you rub your own tight shoulders or neck, trigger points are the areas that may be more sensitive to touch.

Because trigger points usually show up as a noticeable tight spot, and touching or pressing this spot leads to a painful or sensitive reaction, you'll have no trouble finding them. The surefire way to know if you've located a trigger point is to apply firm pressure in a small, localized point. If you press on it and yelp, you can bet you've hit a trigger point.

Trigger points also can cause general pain, tightness or restriction of movement, false heart pain, headaches, neck and jaw pain, tennis elbow, joint pain, restless legs, numbness in the hands and feet, and even what's known as "referred" pain—pain that shows up in a completely different part of the body from the trigger point causing it.

Trigger the Path to Health

When you have a trigger point, your muscle cells and your brain develop communication issues.

Amber Davies, a trigger point specialist and author, describes trigger points as knots in the muscle where the motor nerve enters the belly of the muscle fiber, telling it what to do. The muscle cells are constantly contracted, so they get tired. When this happens, they send a message to the brain saying they are running out of energy and they need some help. But with a trigger point, rather than telling the muscle to relax, the brain just tells it to contract further.

Eventually, the knot becomes so tight that it starts sending pain messages— pain that is often referred to another area of the body.

Trigger points and pain go hand in hand. Returning your muscles to a state of homeostasis is yet another aspect of the Wellness Model of Health™. So let's explore the true negative influence of trigger points and the dramatic impact they can have on your health.

This chapter will discuss trigger points and other problems that result from them, what causes trigger points and their different types, referred pain, trigger point therapy, and how to take your health into your own hands.

Trigger Points Lead to Other Problems

Trigger points, as the name suggests, set a pain cycle in motion. Once you have a trigger point, or several of them, this disrupts your natural state of homeostasis. You will likely alter the way you move, sit, or stand to instinctively protect yourself, just as the muscle is contracting to protect itself. Moving a certain way causes you pain, so you try to avoid it.

Unfortunately, this makes the problem worse. Your body begins to adopt crooked postures that tighten other muscles, leading to additional or worsening existing muscle imbalances. This is one reason some people have both nerve-based back pain caused by muscle imbalances and tissue-based back pain caused by a knot or trigger point within a single muscle.

Bad postures then put pressure on joints and ligaments, further restricting your activities and worsening your overall health. This vicious cycle can come full circle, creating more trigger points and starting the process all over again.

You can see how this quickly leads to lower back pain if you have trigger points anywhere around the lower body. But even more than that, imbalanced postures have implications for the body as a whole.

Remember that, because the fascia connects the entire body, trigger points in one area can cause pain somewhere else. It's not uncommon for a sore neck to be the result of trigger points in the shoulder. In much the same way, fibromyalgia pain—which is noted as pervasive pain throughout the body—is often rooted in a prevalence of trigger points.

To be certain that you're dealing with a trigger point, check for the same hard point on the opposite side of the body. If you find one near the right shoulder blade, for instance, check near the left shoulder blade. If you find a similar hard spot, it's probably a bone, but if you don't, that first one was probably a trigger point.

Trigger point pain in the upper back, shoulders, and neck often can lead to headaches and other ailments as well. To live a healthy, pain-free life, it's critical to treat and relieve trigger points as quickly and thoroughly as possible.

What Causes Trigger Points?

Now you know what's happening, but you still need to know why. While many factors contribute to the development of trigger points, one of the most common is blood circulation that's too slow or restricted—in other words, a deficiency in blood flow.

One major cause of this restricted blood circulation is stress. When you're experiencing an excess of stress, you tend to tense your muscles (reducing blood circulation in those muscles), drink too little water (a deficiency that reduces the blood volume available to clear out toxins in the muscles), eat too much unhealthy food (an excess that causes inflammation that makes trigger points swell), and forget to move around and stretch (a stagnation that reduces blood circulation in your muscles).

These behaviors lead to shallow breathing, which delivers too little oxygen to your muscles—another deficiency. Your excess tension and anxiety lead to decreased blood flow—a stagnation. You can see how all of this ties back to the Wellness Model of Health™.

Without adequate blood flow, the muscle cells in the trigger point areas of your body are unable to activate the relaxation response that makes the trigger point disappear or at least go dormant. This is because the mechanism that allows muscle cells to "let go" requires the oxygen and energy provided by good blood circulation.

Amber Davies told me in an interview that another cause of trigger points is when the muscle is suddenly overloaded. She uses an example of slipping on ice or on water that has spilled on the floor. When you start to slip, suddenly all of your muscles contract. Your arms flail, and your inner thigh muscles and abdominal muscles contract. Those muscles are all working overtime to keep you from falling.

Trigger points also can occur as a result of muscle trauma, muscle strain from repetitive movements or strenuous exercise, muscle imbalances, sitting for long periods, nutritional deficiencies, and more. Unfortunately, once you have a trigger point, it tends to undergo a self-reinforcing cycle—which means it sticks around for a while.

Active and Inactive Trigger Points

Most of us are walking around with trigger points. Just the stresses of living can create them in our bodies over time. Whether or not they cause us pain hinges on whether or not they are "active" at any particular time.

Active trigger points are the ones that feel painful. Dr. Greg Fors, DC, a certified neurologist and author of *Why We Hurt*, calls these active primary trigger points, and describes them as the ones you can find easily, such as by reaching back onto your shoulder blade. These are often treated by practitioners or through self-treatment products, due to their ability to be identified, but it doesn't get rid of the problem completely.

Inactive trigger points, or as Dr. Fors calls them secondary trigger points, don't radiate pain, but may still exist as knots and feel painful if you apply pressure to them. These are formed as a result of the primary trigger points. When they are not removed, they tend to kick off the primary trigger points again and a painful cycle ensues.

After a trigger point has healed, that area of the muscle tends to have a good memory. The trigger point has "branded" it, so to speak, so the next time you experience stress, overwork certain muscles, or fail to drink enough water, that muscle can contract again in the same place, activating the same trigger point as before.

Imagine a ceramic coffee cup. Let's say that one day you accidentally drop it and break the handle. No worries; you use some superglue and seal the handle back on. But that handle now has an old injury. You can bet that if were you to drop the cup again, the handle would break in the very same place.

Trigger points act the same way, particularly if they aren't healed completely. They tend to return again and again, whenever the body is under stress. The best approach is to adopt healing solutions and lifestyle habits that keep trigger points relaxed and dormant—and keep new ones from developing.

Trigger Points and "Referred" Pain

Trigger points can also cause pain in other parts of the body. This is known as "referred" pain. It's as if the trigger point "refers" its pain to some other muscle or area of the body, saying, "Here, you take this message to the brain."

For example, you could be feeling pain in your hips, buttocks, or down your legs, when the actual trigger point is located in your lower back. Trigger points also can refer pain to other trigger points along the same nerve pathways.

So if your health practitioner is not educated in seeking out the cause of the pain, he or she may simply focus on the location of that pain—your legs, for example—while ignoring the fact that the trigger point in your lower back is causing it. That's unfortunate, because then any treatments your practitioner implements will only partially (if at all) help the condition.

Another example is pain in your arm, mid-back, or neck. All of these could be caused by a trigger point in your shoulder. Any treatment that fails to address your shoulder problem is going to be unsuccessful. Therefore, it's important to find the trigger points, wherever they are, and heal them, one by one.

What is Trigger Point Therapy?

What can you do about trigger point pain? Luckily, procedures and devices have been developed to help treat it.

Trigger point therapy is a method by which steady, sustained pressure is applied to the "knotted" area. Such pressure gradually encourages the muscle fibers to relax and release, loosening the twisted places. Since muscles that have trigger points are typically too tight and too short, trigger point therapy encourages elongation and relaxation.

As the fibers return to a more healthy shape, they release all the pent-up toxins that had been trapped there, returning these to the bloodstream where they can be washed away. Blood flow increases through the area, encouraging healing and further waste removal through a return to homeostasis. Eventually, muscle spasms disappear, tension goes away, and the muscle returns to a more normal level of functioning.

This process also creates an overall body release, or "sigh of relief," reducing the pain signals to the brain and alerting your system to restore itself.

This kind of therapy is helpful for any type of pain or illness that originates in trigger points, which can include lower back pain, upper back pain, neck pain, any muscle-based pain, and fibromyalgia—and even some nerve-based pain like sciatica and herniated discs, if the muscles around the nerves are knotted up in trigger points.

Water: Essential to Healing

When you're undergoing treatment for trigger points, it's essential to drink a lot of water. Pressure on the knots in your muscles releases toxin buildup, which means those toxins then become more plentiful in your bloodstream. You need water to flush them out of the body.

Imagine hard water buildup in a humidifier or copper pipe. Once that buildup is broken down into smaller pieces, you need extra water to wash it away. Otherwise, it will continue to linger, and perhaps even build up to become an unhealthy excess in other locations.

If you have a very severe case of trigger point back pain, don't be surprised if, after your first one or two treatments, you feel a little ill. If you had a lot of toxin buildup in your muscles, those toxins will flood your body once released, which can have a physical effect on you. You're essentially releasing months' worth of garbage from your muscles into your bloodstream—ultimately allowing your kidneys to convert the waste into urine.

Drink plenty of water to ensure that these toxin levels don't get so high they make you feel sick.

Three Trigger Point Solutions

The following are three solutions to trigger points and the pros and cons of each: 1) the handheld pressuring device, 2) trigger point massage therapy, and 3) the self-treatment platform.

1. The Handheld Pressuring Device

A popular item on the market is the handheld self-massager, usually a plastic device shaped like a hook or cane, with rounded "balls" on either end and on additional "steps" along the straight edge. These rounded sections are meant to be used to apply pressure to your trigger points. Two examples of this are the "Theracane" and the "Backnobber."

Similar to a back scratcher, this device requires you to do your own work on the areas that are causing you pain. Essentially, you hold the device in your hand, maneuver it to reach the trigger point (usually in your back), and apply pressure, typically in an area no larger than a quarter. The shape of the device gives you some leverage, but you're using your muscles to do the work. You move the ball back and forth across the trigger point, wiggling it a bit to get deeper into the muscle.

The idea is that, after several repeated applications of pressure with the device, your trigger points will loosen up, release toxins, and gradually relieve you of pain.

The good thing about this solution is that it puts you in charge of your own relief. You have the device in your home, where you can use it at your convenience. It's fairly economical—a one-time purchase—and can be used as often as you need without additional cost.

However, these devices can sometimes make your situation worse. Basically, unless you're using the device on your legs, you're asking the same muscles that may be experiencing pain to fix the problem.

For example, if you have a trigger point in the muscle behind your shoulder blade, you have to use that same muscle to maneuver the device and apply pressure to the trigger point. It's like asking a person with a sprained ankle to walk himself to the hospital.

Using this device on any trigger point in any area of your back is going to require the same (or nearby) back muscles to work. If you're not careful, you could be creating more trigger points in muscles that are already overworked, shortened, and inflamed.

Keeping the above in mind, I recommend that you try using a device like this and see how it works for you. While I personally find it to be a great tool, it does require effort to keep your upper-body muscles as relaxed as possible.

2. Trigger Point Massage Therapy

Trigger point massage can be a very effective therapy. It's a form of massage in which the practitioner applies deep pressure to isolated areas of your body— your trigger points.

Trigger point massage is different than regular massage. Instead of implementing longer, sloping movements that lightly pressure the length of your muscles, the therapist will apply targeted, firm, and sustained pressure (about seven to ten seconds) directly on the trigger point. At first, this probably won't feel very good. The trigger point is painful, and pressure will activate that pain—as well as release toxins—both of which can be uncomfortable.

However, if proper pressure is applied on a regular basis, eventually the trigger points will relax and release, and your pain will go away. The pressure physically forces blood circulation into the trigger point area, giving the muscle cells in the trigger point the oxygen and fuel needed to activate the relaxation mechanism.

Trigger point massage is a great solution. The only drawbacks are that it can get very expensive and can take up a considerable amount of your time. One treatment isn't going to do the trick. You need to go back several times to completely release or heal the trigger points—often at least weekly—and since this type of specialty massage typically costs from sixty to a hundred dollars per hour, it can add up in a hurry.

However, there are other solutions that work well, are more convenient, and cost much less.

3. Trigger Point Self-Treatment Platform

There is also a platform that allows you to self-treat your trigger points while keeping your muscles completely relaxed. With these, you simply lie down on a platform that has a number of soft, rubber-tipped "digits" (like fingers) on top, which you can adjust to various positions in order to apply the right amount of pressure in the right place.

You configure this platform to match the trigger points on your back. For example, if you have a trigger point just under your right shoulder blade, you place a pressure bump on the platform in the position where your right shoulder will be when you lie down.

The idea is not to apply pressure to every part of your back, but only to the parts that have trigger points. You position the rubber-tipped pressure bumps where you need them and then lie down on top of them. Gravity takes over.

Because the platform comes with pressure providers of different heights, you can choose the intensity of the pressure. Shorter providers give lighter pressure; longer ones, more intense pressure. This allows you to configure the platform to mirror the location and severity of the trigger points in your back.

There are several advantages to this sort of device. First, it doesn't require sore, irritated muscles to work harder in an effort to gain relief. Second, you're investing once in a device you can use for the rest of your life, so you're saving a significant amount of money. Third, you're putting yourself in charge of your relief, which means you can use the device when it's most convenient for you, and as often as you need it, with minimal hassle.

Finally, it's the sort of solution that gives you immediate feedback. When you lie on a trigger point, you'll know it, because of the sore, numb, or slightly painful reaction in the muscle. If you don't feel that reaction, you can adjust your position on the platform or adjust the pressure providers to a location that will be more effective. It's a very intuitive process that's easy to perform.

Be Your Own Advocate

When it comes to caring for your body, you should always have a hand in your own healing.

Trigger points are problems that we may be able to live with for now, but if we don't address them, they will become much bigger. You need to take responsibility for yourself, because you are your own best advocate, and you are the one who best understands your own excesses, deficiencies, and stagnations. As Amber Davies says, you are the only one who has access to your complete medical file; the only central database is in your own head.

If you can't be your own advocate, then find someone who can. Take a trusted person with you to your appointments to take notes and make sure your questions are answered.

Keeping a pictorial journal is another way to keep on top of your medical issues. Write down a description of your pain. This will help you to track your progress and determine which treatments are working and which aren't as you reestablish a healthy balance. This journaling technique is useful not only in tracking your trigger point pain, but also for any other ailments you might have. Taking this extra step towards self-health can document and establish patterns that you and your doctors wouldn't otherwise see.

Once you've decided to pull the trigger on your own pain relief, you will have one of the most important tools that you need to return your body to homeostasis. But there are even more physical wellness tools at your disposal, and the next one I want to share with you has helped countless people relieve and eliminate severe pain: spinal decompression.

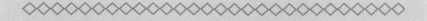

Chapter Review

- Pain and trigger points go hand in hand, and can have a dramatic impact on your health.

- Trigger points can alter the way you move, sit, or stand, which can cause additional imbalance and pain.

- In the upper back, shoulders, and neck, trigger points often lead to headaches and other ailments.

- Stress can cause trigger points by restricting blood circulation to the muscles.

- Trigger points can occur as a result of muscle trauma or strain, repetitive movements, muscle imbalances, sitting for long periods of time, and nutritional deficiencies.

- Active trigger points feel painful; inactive trigger points don't radiate pain, but may still exist as knots and feel painful when you apply pressure to them.

- Trigger points can cause "referred pain" in other parts of the body.

- You can easily "self-treat" your trigger points using inexpensive tools (or even just your bare hands).

Recommended Resources

Why We Hurt: A Complete Physical & Spiritual Guide to Healing Your Chronic Pain by Dr. Gregory Fors. Dr. Fors's book offers more detailed information on pain and trigger points.

Trigger Point Self-Treatment System

The Healthy Back Institute recommends a few different trigger point self-treatment systems. Using these systems is one of the easiest ways to get deep-pressure massage in the comfort of your own home. Learn more at www.losethebackpain.com/triggerpiontselftreatment.html.

CHAPTER 9:

Spinal Compression: The Backbone of Health

The Backbone of Your Health

I've told you how muscle imbalances can lead to pain, and how pain caused by trigger points can cascade throughout your entire body. Another common source of pain and other health problems stems from the spine.

Our spines are part of the big picture when it comes to managing excess, deficiency, and stagnation. They support the weight of our entire body. They also house and protect our nerves, allowing for the free flow of communication and information throughout the body. Unfortunately, with so many moving pieces that have the potential to disrupt our overall state of homeostasis, many problems can result from spinal misalignment or an inflamed spine.

I've already covered the impact that muscle imbalances and trigger points can have on your spinal alignment, as well as the influence they can have on your overall health. What I haven't discussed yet is how the health of the spine, specifically the discs between the bones, can likewise have a huge impact on your health as a whole.

So here is a trivia question for you: How is your spine like a balloon?

The spine is made up of a series of bones called vertebrae that are stacked one on top of the other. In between these bones are doughnut-shapes discs—gel-like structures that are filled mostly with water that serve as the body's shock absorbers.

Now imagine a water balloon. If you were to squish one side with your fist, all the water in the balloon would form a bulge at the other side. Keep pressing and eventually you could force the other end of the balloon to burst.

The discs in your spine operate much the same way as that water balloon. As muscle imbalances—and gravity—apply uneven pressure on a disc, the disc bulges to one side. As you go about your day, gravity presses down on your discs, causing the water inside them to slowly squeeze out. In fact, measurements taken have shown that most people are slightly shorter at the end of the day than they were at the beginning—by as much as three-quarters of an inch!

When your disc bulges like that water balloon, it develops a herniation. This bulge then often comes in contact with a nerve, which is what many doctors believe causes the sharp, radiating pain of this condition. Eventually, if the problem is not corrected, the disc can burst, losing its water content and its ability to absorb any shock at all. Moreover, spinal problems like compression can lead to a host of chronic illnesses.

Even if we don't have muscle imbalances adding to the issue, which we all do, gravity by itself creates a daily compression on our spines. Fortunately, the spinal discs reabsorb water while we sleep (as long as we're not dehydrated), so we start the day again at close to our regular height. However, over the years, our discs lose their ability to "re-inflate," so we grow a little shorter by the time we become seniors.

Luckily, there are options to help combat spinal compression, such as inversion therapy. In addition to helping reverse the excess compression caused by gravity, inversion therapy has many added benefits. It's important to note that in order for it to be a successful and safe option for you, certain guidelines must be followed.

This chapter will discuss spinal compression, inversion therapy and its various benefits, and when you need to do it, as well as how to use it to find relief from back pain caused by spinal compression.

What Is Inversion Therapy?

As the name states, inversion therapy actually "inverts" the body to an upside down position. There are several ways this can be performed, but the most common is by using what's called an inversion table.

An inversion table sits on a swivel and is made for you to lie on. Think of a seesaw with a bed on it—only the midpoint of the seesaw is much higher, so if you lean all the way forward, you're fully upright, and if you lean all the way back, you're upside down.

The idea behind inversion therapy is to reverse the effects of gravity. Since we live on Earth, we're all subjected to the force of gravity on a day-to-day basis. Our muscles and bones help us stand up against it, but over the years, it tends to wear us down a bit—particularly the spine, which is the center of our upright posture.

How Does It Help?

Inversion therapy reverses the excess compression caused by gravity—and in part, by muscle imbalances. In essence, it reverses the pressure on the spine. Instead of compressing your discs and making you shorter, inversion therapy—by allowing you to hang upside down—actually stretches out the spine and the muscles that support both it and torso, giving the discs room to reabsorb fluids and move back into their proper positions, eliminating pressure on nearby nerves.

With the increased spaces between the vertebrae that inversion therapy creates, discs are suddenly relieved of pressure and have room to breathe, so to speak. Even the slightest increase in spacing can create a mild suction, which can encourage a bulging disc to return to its normal position. In essence, creating this space gives the disc the room it needs to heal.

If you picture that balloon again, it's like taking your fist off one end and allowing the air inside to fill up the entire area once again.

What does this mean to you? Pain relief. If a disc is pressing on a nerve, inversion therapy will often relieve that pressure, easing pain almost immediately.

According to many clinical studies, inversion therapy is one of the most effective and fastest ways to increase space between your vertebrae. Participants have reported that their back pain, pain that had plagued them for decades, totally disappeared with just a few minutes of inversion therapy.

Other cases completely reversed themselves after just a week of inversion therapy—ten minutes a day of hanging upside down. If you need to get back to work and you suspect a herniated disc could be the source of your pain, inversion therapy may be the best way to recover.

And in case you doubt the effectiveness of inversion therapy, a study conducted by Newcastle University found that sufferers of back pain who underwent inversion therapy were 75 percent less likely to require back surgery!

Benefits beyond the Back

Though increasing space between the vertebrae is one of the biggest benefits of inversion therapy, it's definitely not the only one. Let's take a look at several other benefits.

Improves circulation. Turning the body upside down, for your blood, is like taking a road that normally climbs uphill and making it go downhill. In other words, where the blood usually had to travel up, it now heads down, and vice versa. Suddenly it's easier for the blood to get to certain areas that are usually a challenge to reach—particularly the upper back, neck, and head. This makes it easier for parts of the body to have easier access to the nutrients and oxygen they need.

Lengthens muscles and ligaments. Inverting the body has a natural stretching effect on many of your muscles and ligaments. You can feel this while it's happening. Pitch yourself upside down for even a moment and you'll feel some of the muscles in your back, legs, and hips pulling toward the ground. Since these muscles are usually pulled in the opposite direction by gravity, inversion therapy helps counteract this, pulling your muscles in the other direction and increasing flexibility.

Relieves joints. Point your head toward the ground and, instantly, knee, hip, ankle, and other joints experience a gentle "opening." Similar to the way inversion therapy eases pressure on the spine, it does the same to weight-bearing joints that are typically loaded all the time, every day. With the absence of pressure, the joints get momentary relief, during which they, like the discs in the spine, gradually open up and "breathe." This effect can be felt for hours after the therapy, in joints that feel more springy and supple.

Improves posture. Though inversion therapy will not correct muscle imbalances, it may help a crooked spine to realign itself. By using the power of gravity to pull in the opposite direction, inversion therapy encourages the spine to resume its normal posture.

It's like pulling on the bottom of a wrinkled shirt to straighten it out. Gravity pulls the spine toward your head. Given enough time (through repeat treatments), the vertebrae can line back up. When you stand upright again, you'll feel the effects and enjoy better posture. If you combine this therapy with muscle balance therapy, you'll be more likely to maintain that improved body position.

Maintains your height. We would all like to maintain our stature as we get older. Inversion therapy helps counteract the typical wearing down of the spine over the years, helping us avoid the shrinkage associated with old age. Discs that have been ground down over time get a "breather" and a chance to reabsorb fluid so they can regain their shock-absorbing capacity. It's these same discs that, when worn down, contribute to that hunched-back posture that plagues many older people.

Increases mental alertness. Some authorities believe that increasing oxygen and blood flow to the brain can help maintain mental sharpness. Since this is such an important goal for seniors—as evidenced by all the sales of mental-support supplements—such a benefit could be very welcome.

Helps in workout recovery. Running, cycling, and other aerobic activities can actively compress the spine, oftentimes in uneven ways. One-sided sports like tennis, racquetball, and golf can pull the spine out of alignment because of the repeated twisting motions associated with these activities. With regular inversion therapy, any misalignments between the vertebrae often are self-corrected.

Is It Safe?

Some people may have heard that inversion therapy can increase the chance of having a stroke. I think this is the unfortunate result of misinformation. Yes, there was a study published in 1983 by Dr. Steven A. Goldman in which he observed that inverted patients experienced an increase in blood pressure. The media jumped on the story, warning people that inversion therapy could lead to stroke.

What they didn't report as widely was that two years later Dr. Goldman recanted his position, stating, "New research shows that you are at no more of a stroke risk hanging upside down than if you are exercising right-side up." He said that the media's warnings about inversion therapy were "grossly inflated."

Further research actually discovered that the body has built-in ways to prevent any damage from hanging upside down. Unfortunately, this news wasn't as exciting, so few people ever heard it, and many remained concerned about using this very beneficial treatment.

Of course, you should be in basic good health if you're going to try inversion therapy. If you have high blood pressure, heart disease, an eye condition, are pregnant, or have had fusion surgery or a knee or hip replacement, you should check with your doctor before trying inversion therapy. Additionally, if you have bone weakness, recent fractures or skeletal implants, are using anti-coagulants, or are obese, you will also want to check with your doctor prior to seeking this kind of treatment.

That said, research shows that this therapy is as safe as most daily activities.

What Is the Best Way to Do It?

Though "gravity boots" were popular in the 1980s, the most common way to invert today is by using an inversion table. There are a wide variety of these on the market. So what do you need to look for?

First, you should invest in a quality inversion table—one that's going to last and that has the proper safety features. There are a lot of companies who make these, and many of them skimp on quality to bring their prices down. If you're hanging upside down, you want something that's going to support you, time after time. You don't want to save a few bucks just to land on your head! Look for a table that's adjustable, safe, durable, and convenient for using in your home.

A process that includes a gradual increase of the angle of inversion, as well as a gradual increase of time spent upside down, is best for relieving back pain. A good user's manual or video guide can help you set up such a process for yourself, increasing your odds of success.

Equipment Specifics

When you're in pain, you don't want to contort your body to get inverted. Look for an extended handle on the table that will let you lock your ankles securely in place without having to "touch your toes" and injure your back in your quest to help your back.

When inverted, your weight will be supported by your ankles. So for comfort's sake, make sure you get a table with foam-based ankle grips. These reduce the amount of pressure on your ankles while ensuring that you're still secure and safe. And your ankles will thank you for not using a hard molded variety.

Those who are new to inversion almost universally have the same two questions. A good inversion table will answer both of those questions for you.

1)   How can I control how far (upside) down I go?

Your inversion table should have a simple mechanism to allow you to set the maximum angle you want to invert before you start. Usually, this comes in the form of a tether strap that allows you to select a particular angle.

Remember—you do not need to go completely upside down to get the full benefit of inversion! Between twenty and thirty degrees is enough to gently stretch and relax tight muscles, while sixty degrees takes the entire load of gravity off your spine.

2)   How can I make sure I can get back up?

Getting back up from an inverted position is super easy once you know how. But the first time or two might be a little nerve wracking if you forget the "trick" to it. So for ease of mind, make sure to get a table with big, easy to reach handles you can use to help yourself up if you ever need them.

If your table doesn't come with at least a one-year warranty, keep looking. That simply means the manufacturer knows they're selling junk that will break in less than a year if you use it every day.

Besides the regular warranty, look for a satisfaction guarantee that allows you to try the table out at home and return it if you're not satisfied. There's no point in getting stuck with a piece of equipment that won't work for you.

Don't Want to Hang Upside Down?

If you have reservations about this type of therapy, there are other spinal decompression options available that can help you realize similar results.

Unless you are made of money, you will likely want to skip the expensive spinal decompression machines found at chiropractic offices. They will produce a similar result, but the pain in your wallet may overcome the pain relief in your back.

There are other innovations on the market that can give most of the benefits of inversion without the full, upside down posture.

At the Healthy Back Institute, I've heard from a number of customers that they need something that accommodates their lessened range of motion. To this end, we now supply an inversion table that allows the user to start in a seated position. This becomes more like starting in a recliner, and then continuing back until the benefits of inverted decompression are realized. Of course, this still turns you on your head!

Getting Started

I suggest inverting for one to three minutes, one to three times per day at only a slight inversion for the first week or two. As you become more comfortable with inverting, gradually adjust the amount of time and degree of inversion you use.

Remember this rule of thumb: always listen to your body. If you feel uncomfortable, simply stop inverting and try again later. Remember that even too much of a healthy practice is still an excess under the Wellness Model of Health™.

The degree of inversion you choose affects how long you need to invert for the same results. For example, the shallower the degree, the longer the inversion time needed. The higher the degree of inversion, the shorter the inversion time needed.

Try oscillating, or slowly rocking back and forth to and from the inverted position. During this movement you'll invert for twenty to thirty seconds, then return upright for twenty to thirty seconds and repeat the rhythm.

Many doctors recommend this movement pattern during inversion as it helps stimulate the circulation of blood and lymph for faster healing.

Again, you do not need to fully invert to start to capture the health benefits of inversion. Take your time and work up to sixty degrees for maximum benefit. After you are comfortable at sixty degrees of inversion for a few weeks, go ahead and try a full inversion if you want—but start out for only thirty seconds. My experience is that 95 percent of all discomfort comes from trying to invert too much, too fast, for too long. Again, listen to your body and take your time.

Inversion Exercises

Movement while inverted is particularly helpful for decompressing the spine while increasing your mobility and flexibility. Once you're comfortable inverting, try introducing these gentle stretches and exercises to your inversion routine.

Lower Back

You may perform gentle stretching exercises to help move the muscles and connective tissues in your lower back area.

In partial inversion, try rotating gently from side-to-side or slowly rocking your pelvis forward and backward.

If you have worked up to full inversion, abdominal exercises (sit-ups, crunches) can be beneficial for your lower back, since strong abdominal muscles are important for proper posture. Also try a gentle back extension by placing your hands behind your head on the bed frame and pushing your body in an arch away from the table.

Upper Back

Many people experience upper back pain as a result of stress and muscle tension. The key to relieving this pain is to totally relax while inverting. Try deep breathing exercises while inverted. Partner work can be very helpful— nothing is more relaxing than an inverted back and shoulder massage!

Movement is also very beneficial. Try rounding your shoulders forward and pushing them back. Then stretch one arm at a time across your torso to extend those upper back muscles for a gentle stretch.

Neck

Similar to your upper back, movement can be beneficial for neck pain. Try rotating your head from one side to the other. Partner massages to the base of your head and back of your neck are very relaxing (do not apply pressure to the front of the neck).

Try adding gentle inverted traction to your neck by resting your arms behind your head at the base of your skull (don't pull, just add the weight of your arms).

Spinal Relief

The bottom line is that your normal day-to-day living puts stress on your spine, and that plays a big role in the excess, deficiency, and stagnation of many other things in your health. The good news is that you can incorporate inversion therapy into your routine and get relief—along with many other additional benefits—when you work toward physical balance in the Complete Healing Formula™.

Remember, the positive impact of spinal decompression stretches far beyond your spine itself. You'll also experience all kinds of cardiovascular improvements, joint pain relief, and the other benefits mentioned in this chapter.

Once you know the basics, inversion therapy is a safe and simple solution. If it's done properly, your back and your whole body will thank you.

Both the physical and mental tools I've shown you as part of the Wellness Model of Health™ over the past several chapters can be summed up under a single nature: energy. When you understand how both of these frequencies work, you can use them to enhance health and wellness in your life. The next chapter will cover the different modalities of these energy pathways.

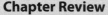

Chapter Review

- Our spines support the weight of our entire body, and they house and protect our nerves. The health of your spine can have a huge impact on your overall health.

- Spinal compression is caused by gravity and muscle imbalances, and it can lead to a host of chronic illnesses.

- Inversion therapy inverts the body to an upside down position, relieving spinal compression.

- The benefits of spinal decompression include: improved circulation, lengthened muscles and ligaments, joint relief, improved posture, height maintenance, increased mental alertness, and improved workout recovery.

- When beginning inversion therapy, start by inverting for one to three minutes, one to three times per day at only a slight inversion for the first week or two. As you become more comfortable with inverting, gradually adjust the amount of time and degree of inversion you use.

Recommended Resources

Inversion Therapy

You can learn more about inversion therapy, and find out more about which tools will best suit your needs, at http://www.losethebackpain.com/inversion3.html.

CHAPTER 10:

Energy Medicine: Health Secret or New-Age Hoax?

A Force for Health

You are already an energy expert. You might not realize it, but you are.

As you go about your day, you constantly use and sense energy within yourself and in the world around you. What you might not realize is that if you take the time to harness those energies to restore homeostasis to your mind, body, and diet, they can have a powerful and positive impact on your health and well-being.

We're all accustomed to the fact that we need to consume food to generate the energy to move. That's why food is measured in calories. Calories are simply a measurement of energy. But the importance and presence of energy aren't limited to the food we eat and the activities we practice.

Everything in the universe is made up of energy, and this energy exists in many varieties and vibrates at specific frequencies. There is dense energy, loose energy, erratic energy, and calm energy, as well as both high and low frequencies.

The human body, too, is nothing if not a physical body constructed of energetic vibrations. Considering this, you can see how energy encompasses the physical, mental, and dietary components of the Complete Healing Formula™ combined: all three of these things deal in different frequencies of energy.

All aspects of health and well-being are tied to energetic frequencies. If we think of energy in the form of frequencies, like a radio, we can start to see a big piece of our problem—especially as it relates to pain. Most of us who suffer chronic pain and illness only get the "pain and sickness channel" and keep ourselves "tuned in" to it 24/7. In this way, we get stuck on the "pain and sickness frequency," and our suffering becomes needlessly prolonged.

But a radio doesn't have to stay on just one channel, and neither do our bodies. It just depends on what we dial into. If you tune in to an opera channel on your radio, you will get opera, not country music. If you dial your mother on the cell phone, you won't get cousin Betty. If you say bad things about people, you will lose friends. "You reap what you sow," is a good example of the power of attraction, the power of like energy meeting like energy.

You've probably noticed how some people are more upbeat and happy than others, and how that attitude can be infectious. The mental energy of these individuals creates a mood or atmosphere that, if you let it, can rub off on you a bit. Or consider the effect of the energy frequencies you feel when you walk into a funeral parlour. The mood there is far different than it is at, for instance, a sporting event.

To make this a little more concrete, think about a time when you were very tired. You may have had trouble thinking, remembering names, or enjoying a usually pleasant experience. The literal lack of physical energy caused by poor sleep created a lack of mental energy, so your mind was vibrating at a lower frequency during that experience—a perfect example of how the mental and physical unite under the concept of energy.

Similarly, if your physical energy is blocked or sluggish, you will experience aches and pains such as sciatica, headaches, fibromyalgia, and other things. In short, low frequency equals low function and poor health; high frequency equals high function and good health. These excesses, deficiencies, and stagnations need to be addressed with the Wellness Model of Health™.

You must change your energetic frequency to feel better and live better. This chapter will show you how.

Your "Energetic" Body

Traditional cultures around the world built their healing models on correcting energetic imbalances—excesses, deficiencies, and stagnations—in the body. Dr. Wiley investigated these cultures in detail during his research around the globe. He found that the role of Shamans in Siberia, Alaska, and Southeast Asia was to eradicate "bad spirits" (i.e., negative energy) from the body to restore physical or mental health in those suffering.

The entire foundation of Chinese and Indian healing practices was built on the premise of energy systems and pathways in the body that, when blocked, cause pain and disease. Clearing these channels or centers of blocked energy (e.g., toxins, spasms) is what restores health to the ill and offers relief to the pain sufferer.

The most common term used to describe human energy is an "aura." This is a general term used to describe the color, mood, or quality of five overlapping energy layers. These layers of energy (or energy bodies) refer to the spiritual, mental, emotional, etheric, and physical energies that make up humans.

Energy is developed, stored, and moved in the body through the adrenals, organs, chakra centers, and meridian pathways. There is a saying in Traditional Chinese Medicine that speaks to why we experience pain: "Where there is energy blockage, there is pain. Where energy moves freely, there is no pain."

The key to pain relief and lasting health, then, is to open the energy channels, raise your vibration frequency, and keep your energy moving at a constant rate of homeostasis at all times. There are a number of alternative therapies that Dr. Wiley unearthed in his book, *Arthritis Reversed,* whose primary function is to do just that. With his permission, I have listed these therapies for you below.

Energy Therapies

Polarity Therapy

Like several other energy medicine methodologies, polarity therapy views the human body as comprising "life energy." However, polarity therapy takes the view that the energy body is in a state of constant "pulsation," with positive and negative poles and a neutral position.

These poles and position form a kind of energetic "template" along the body. A practitioner can apply touch and pressure to this energetic template to alter the pulsations and encourage pain relief and better general states of health.

While it shares common ideas with acupressure and QiGong, Dr. Wiley found that polarity therapy is more aligned with Indian Ayurvedic medicine and modern osteopathic and chiropractic theories of the body.

When people have gone through the complete series of acupuncture or QiGong treatments recommended by their practitioner, and have not found substantial relief, polarity therapy may be the next best modality to embrace. Oftentimes, a person's polarity (positive/negative energy poles) is reversed, and one or more polarity sessions can correct this.

Quantum Touch®

In terms of hands-on energy work, the new kid on the block is Quantum Touch®. It is both a method for individuals to work on themselves and for practitioners to work on those in need of its healing potential. It does this through simple methods that amplify and appropriately channel life force energy. This process helps the body facilitate its own healing process.

Quantum Touch®'s claim to relieve chronic pain was put to the test through an eight-week pilot study where the investigators used twelve volunteer adult patients (men and women, ranging in age from eighteen to sixty-four) who were randomly selected and assigned to an experimental and control group of six volunteers in each group. Both groups were blindfolded and received hands-on touch; however, only the experimental group was given the Quantum Touch® energy.

As Dr. Wiley reports, what was made very clear through this research is that Quantum Touch® healing is effective and has a positive impact on clients in the area of chronic musculoskeletal pain. This holistic modality, like others before it, can now offer itself to the world of health and wellness as a viable method of pain management, with documented evidence of its impact and effectiveness.

Reiki

Reiki is a Japanese energy practice used to reduce stress and induce relaxation to help promote the free-flow of energy in the body. To share the benefits of Reiki, practitioners use both non-touch and "laying on of hands" techniques.

Reiki practitioners lay their hands on or near patients in various configurations modeled on powerful, ancient Tibetan and Chinese healing symbols. It is believed that recreating these symbols on the body will allow "God's energy" to flow from the Universe, through the practitioner, and into the patient.

Because this energy vibrates at a high frequency, it will lift the low energy of the sufferer to relieve pain and illness.

Reiki has become a popular healing modality among nurses in hospitals. The patient does not have to be awake for them to administer a few minutes of healing touch. It may be the easiest of the energy healing systems to find a practitioner, and it also feels really good.

However, Reiki seems to have the least corrective benefits. It's good for relaxation and acute symptomatic relief, but not as effective for long-term relief based on being a truly corrective body therapy.

Jin Shin Jyutsu

Similar to its Chinese cousins, Jin Shin Jyutsu aims to balance the physical and mental energies in the body. It views the body as being composed of a trinity of energy pathways that, when functioning properly, harmonize mind, body and spirit.

Jin Shin Jyutsu's healing ability is rooted in manipulating and opening twenty-six energy points, known as the "safety energy factors." When activated through finger pressure, these points unblock stagnant energy, relieve tension and allow energy to flow freely in the body. Like acupressure, patients can both receive treatment from a practitioner, or they can learn self-pressure methods to use in regulating their own energy centers.

QiGong Therapy

QiGong refers to specific health exercises or techniques for regulating the body, mind, and breath. These involve visualization, movement, posture, and self-massage to effect interior balance and, in turn, positive changes in health.

Dr. Wiley found that regular practice of QiGong aids in regulating the functions of the central nervous system. Along with exercising and controlling one's mind and body, QiGong influences one's physical states and pathological conditions.

At the same time, the practice of QiGong produces latent energy within the human body, enabling the practitioner to use this to their fullest potential.

Regular practice increases the body's ability to adapt to and defend against the natural and physical environment that we live in.

The primary use of QiGong today is to improve one's health, thus extending life. This is known as medical or healing QiGong and has three subdivisions:

1) Applied clinical therapy, where a Chinese doctor emits (projects) his own *qi* into a patient's body to effect a cure;

2) Self-regulating exercises, performed by a person who chooses a QiGong program and practices the exercises over a period of at least one hundred days to improve his or her own health;

3) A combination of clinical QiGong treatments from a doctor and an individual's personal self-regulating QiGong training program. Within the self-practice method, exercises are done in any combination of three techniques: static postures, slow movements, and meditation and breathing exercises.

Acupuncture and Acupressure

Acupuncture is no longer the backroom healing art it was once thought to be. On the contrary, not only is it a household word, but it is extremely popular among sports competitors and women in their forties and fifties. What's more, mainstream medical doctors are increasingly expanding their own practices to offer acupuncture in their offices.

Still, many people are still leery of this five-thousand-year-old tradition. They wonder if it is real or just new-age hype. The World Health Organization (WHO) has vetted this ancient Chinese healing tradition and announced that acupuncture is suitable for treating the following conditions:

- *Ear, Nose and Throat Disorders*: toothaches, pain after tooth extraction, gingivitis, acute or chronic otitis, acute sinusitis, acute rhinitis, nasal catarrh, and acute tonsillitis.

- *Respiratory Disorders*: asthma, bronchitis, colds, and allergies.

- *Gastrointestinal Disorders*: esophageal and cardio spasm, hiccup, gastroptosis, acute or chronic gastritis, sour stomach, chronic duodenal ulcers, acute or chronic colitis, acute bacillary dysentery, constipation, diarrhea, and paralytic ileus.

- *Eye Disorders*: acute conjunctivitis, central retinitis, nearsightedness (in children), and cataracts.

- *Neurological and Muscular Disorders*: headaches, migraines, trigeminal neuralgia, facial paralysis (within the first three to six months), post-stroke paresis, peripheral neuritis, neurological bladder dysfunction, bed wetting, intercostal neuralgia, cervical syndrome, frozen shoulder, tennis elbow, sciatica, low back pain, and osteoarthritis.

In other words, acupuncture is an effective treatment for a whole host of medical conditions.

Acupressure is the non-invasive and non-needle-using offspring of acupuncture, the therapy where thin needles are inserted into the skin to correct energetic imbalances. Both work on the same theory, and in both cases, the practitioner will either "needle" or apply finger pressure to specific points (acupoints) on the body. Using a correct "prescription" of points, the practitioner can in effect change the energy in a patient, open their channels, and help their energy move more freely.

Acupuncture and acupressure are both widely practiced today and worth looking into. They have been around for five thousand years and have helped millions of people. Acupuncture needles work like antennae, pulling bioelectric energy from the atmosphere into the body to correct energy imbalances within the body's meridian channels.

Frequency Specific Microcurrent (FSM) Therapy

Frequency-specific microcurrent (FSM) therapy treats myofascial neuropathic pain, reducing inflammatory cytokines (polypeptide regulators). In other words, it helps reduce trigger points and fascial constrictions that cause pain, as well as reducing sensations like "pins and needles," coldness or burning, and numbness or itching caused by a damaged or diseased sensory system, as is common in arthritis.

Dr. Wiley explains that FSM is a non-invasive therapy that requires the use of a two-channel microamperage current device that can be purchased online. This treatment requires two separate channels of voltage (13Hz and 396Hz) to be connected to the patient while attempting to move their affected limbs to their utmost range of motion. Clinical studies show that these specific frequencies, when used simultaneously, can effectively treat nerve and muscle pain, reduce inflammation, and clear scar tissue.

Other frequencies help reduce the pain associated with kidney stones, and aid in the healing of asthma, liver dysfunction, irritable bowel syndrome (IBS), and other conditions.

Pulsed Electromagnetic Frequency (PEMF) Therapy

For many, the idea that we are influenced by such a thing as harmful electromagnetic frequency (EMF) smog has never crossed their minds. If you can't see it, it doesn't exist, right?

Wrong. This smog is all around us, every day, everywhere we go. It originates from the frequencies of cell towers, cell and cordless phones, high-definition televisions, laptop computers, microwaves, electrical appliances, computers, fluorescent lighting, Bluetooth devices, Wi-Fi installations, more than two thousand satellites used for GPS, TV, and radio communications, and especially in our vehicles.

EMFs are making us sick and, worse, slowly killing us by breaking down the very structure of our cells. There is no escaping it.

Martin Blank, PhD, of Columbia University says, "Cells in the body react to low level EMFs and produce a biochemical stress response. Our safety standards are inadequate. People need to sit up and pay attention . . . New research is suggesting that nearly all of the human plagues which emerged in the twentieth century, including leukemia in children, female breast cancer, malignant melanomas, immune system disorders, asthma, and others, can be tied in some way to our use of electricity."

How does that affect us from a biological standpoint? As Dr. Wiley explains, in a nutshell, each of our cells is surrounded by a cell membrane. Embedded in the cell membrane are numerous proteins that act as receptors for various molecules, including enzymes. These receptors translate the positive and negative signals on the cell's exterior into its interior, and these signals then trigger various biological processes.

When we're affected by external electromagnetic fields, the high-speed positive/negative polarity switching within these fields, from hundreds to millions of times per second, interferes with our cells' internal signalling process. Basically, it confuses them and they become paralyzed.

Fortunately, a product recently permitted into the United States claims it can reverse this damage in only eight minutes, if used two to three times a day. It's called the MRS2000, and it's a German-engineered medical device that uses pulsed, healthy EMFs to counter the debilitating effects of today's EMF smog and help bring people to optimal health.

It turns out that, much like the discovery of both good and bad cholesterol, certain EMFs are actually good for us. In fact, we can't live without them. As a result, much research has gone into refining pulsed EMF therapy and the results are impressive.

Paul Rosch, MD, of New York Medical College, described it like this: "While EMFs are responsible for quite a bit of damage, don't throw the baby out with the bathwater. Pulsed electromagnetic frequency (PEMF) therapies have been shown to be beneficial for stress related disorders, for anxiety, insomnia, arthritis, depression and more. They also may be safer and more effective than drugs."

Thousands of clinical studies are proving its value, and PEMF therapy is beginning to get the recognition it deserves. In some ways, it sounds similar to the zapping discovered by Dr. Clark that I addressed in an earlier chapter. While experts may not all agree on what EMF exposure levels cause what health issues, the evidence out there suggests we would be foolish not to apply the precautionary principle and reduce our exposure.

Earthing and Grounding

Another energy pathway that is gaining ground is earthing and grounding. Dr. Jim Oschman, author of *Energy Medicine: The Scientific Basis*, has worked for nearly a decade on earthing or grounding, a technique that seeks to connect the body to the earth. He has learned that humans need to make conductive contact with the surface of the earth.

It turns out that the development of plastic and rubber shoe soles has resulted in a major disconnect between us and Mother Nature. It's Dr. Oschman's view that this has had serious consequences for our health. He says that people are rediscovering the healing energies of the earth by simply putting their feet in seawater and walking barefoot on the grass.

According to Dr. Oschman, various technologies are being developed that bring the benefit of the earth's surface right into your home. There are conductive sheets you can buy that have silver fibers. You can put these sheets on your mattress and then connect them to a wire on a rod stuck in the ground outside your bedroom. Dr. Oschman says this helps those with insomnia sleep better. They have less pain because the electrons from the earth are great antioxidants and relieve inflammation in the body.

There is also footwear specifically designed with a small conductive plug at the ball of your foot. When you're walking outside, this conductive plug connects you to the earth. Even if you're walking on cement, it acts as a good conductor and you will feel a difference. Not only can your pain and inflammation be dramatically reduced, this will happen immediately.

Solutions like these are simple and don't require any extra time and effort on your part, but the results can be life-changing.

Energy Medicine

As Dr. Wiley points out in *Arthritis Reversed*, healing and pain relief do not have one-size-fits-all solutions. Energy medicine, like other treatments and therapies discussed in this book, is about addressing excesses, deficiencies, and stagnations. It's about helping the body to heal and not just masking the symptoms. If you view pain as your body's way of telling you something needs to be done, by taking away the pain, you also take away the chance to get to the root of it.

Energy medicine treatments are mild and don't come with the unpleasant side effects that result from many traditional treatments. Add this lack of side effects to their high effectiveness, and this makes energy medicine treatments a winning combination.

The individualistic approach to medicine that most alternative healthcare practitioners use is more effective. This is because they are taking the time to get all the information from you, the patient, so they can help you make the best decisions. They're looking at the big picture. The other bonus here is that you don't have treatments—especially prescriptions—forced on you.

While once thought to be mystical, the science behind energy medicine makes sense if you really think about it. Tap into natural resources, both your own and the earth's, to restore your energy balance and free yourself from pain.

You are now thoroughly equipped to handle both the mental and physical components of the Complete Healing Formula™. But I still have one more key piece of the health puzzle to cover: diet. The next few chapters will take you through everything you need to know about what you put into your body, starting with toxic and moldy foods.

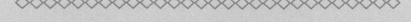

Chapter Review

- You are constantly using and sensing energy within yourself and in the world around you.

- All aspects of health are tied to energetic frequencies. Low-frequency energy results in low function and poor health; high-frequency energy creates high function and good health.

- Energy is developed, stored, and moved in the body through the adrenals, organs, chakra centers, and meridian pathways.

- Different types of energy therapies include: polarity therapy, Quantum Touch®, Reiki, Jin Shin Jyutsu, QiGong, acupuncture and acupressure, frequency specific microcurrent (FSM) therapy, pulsed electromagnetic frequency (PEMF) therapy, and earthing and grounding.

- Energy treatments can be more effective than traditional treatments and have fewer side effects.

Recommended Resources

Arthritis Reversed by Dr. Mark Wiley

You can get a detailed explanation of many of the energy therapies covered in this chapter in Dr. Mark Wiley's book, *Arthritis Reversed* at www.arthritisbookfree.com.

Energy Medicine: The Scientific Basis by Dr. Jim Oschman

To learn more about energy pathways, I recommend Dr. Jim Oshman's book, *Energy Medicine: The Scientific Basis.* You can learn more about his work at www.energyresearch.us.

Live Pain Free Membership

Energy therapies rarely get a fair shake in modern media coverage. I share details and new developments about this important subject regularly with my Live Pain Free family. Join and keep up to speed at losethebackpain.com/membership.

CHAPTER 11:

The Hidden Dangers Lurking In Your Food

Raise the Red Flag

People are beginning to understand that the quality of their food impacts the quality of their lives awakening to the dangers in many of the foods and drinks that comprise our modern diet. However, this knowledge, while it helps form the foundation of a better way of eating, doesn't go far enough.

It's not enough to simply avoid fast food and other clearly "unhealthy" foods. We must be vigilant about what we are consuming and where it came from to truly find the balance we need within our diets. In the upcoming chapters, I'll cover several aspects of the health dangers in our food and water. Here, I'll explore the toxic invaders in our food and water supply that are crippling modern health.

Lurking in the Water

Few doubt the positive impact that water treatment has brought to the modern world. In developed areas, with access to clean water, diseases such as cholera and dysentery are a thing of the past—an accomplishment of great importance for sure! Yet this development owes much of its success to chemicals that are posing an entirely new threat to modern society.

Dr. Clark's research raised my awareness to the presence of certain chemicals in water that are flooding our bodies with new, toxic invaders. The addition of chlorine and other chemicals to most public water supplies puts five immunosuppressants directly into our bodies. These toxins—azo dyes, asbestos, benzene, heavy metals, and PCBs—were found in every one of her cancer patients. To avoid these toxins, you need to know a little more about them and how they end up in our food and water supplies.

As I touched in a previous chapter, heavy metals include substances such as mercury, cadmium, lead, and nickel, along with a few other toxic lighter metals like aluminum and titanium. These make a regular appearance in our drinking water. Additionally, they commonly appear in soft drinks, toothpastes, and even in dental fillings and cutlery. Consumption of these immunosuppressants is common for most of us unless we take specific care to avoid them.

Azo dyes, although carcinogenic, are also frequently found in our water supply due to the chlorination process. In addition, they are included in pesticides, and therefore regularly ride along on commercially sprayed vegetables.

Although we have been told that asbestos has been removed from our environment, that is far from the truth. This substance is still frequently used in conveyor and packaging machinery, where this carcinogen can fly right into our water or onto our food during production.

While benzene is a chemical that our bodies can handle in small amounts, it nonetheless wreaks havoc on our systems when we take in too much of it. Benzene is present in coffee, petroleum jellies, lubricants, and even untested supplements. Since it impedes blood cell development, its impact on our health and ability to heal is self-evident.

Least surprising of all is the presence of PCBs (polychlorinated biphenyls) in chlorinated water, as the chlorination process directly adds these toxins to the water. It is also found in most water bottles as a part of the plastic itself. Unless plastic packaging specifically notes that it is made of "high density polyethylene 2 (HDPE 2)," it is filled with this carcinogenic toxin.

Dr. Clark's research showed her that there were different types of chlorine present in her cancer patients and her non-cancer patients alike. The chlorine approved by the US National Science Foundation contains ferricyanide, which has been shown by Dr. Clark's research to cause other serious diseases, but not cancer.

Yet the chlorine that Dr. Clark says develops cancer does contain potassium ferrocyanide. The difference between these two chemicals may look minor, but that single letter of difference between the two names has dangerous repercussions. People often get confused when presented with safety information on these toxins; ferrocyanide and ferricyanide are two different components, even though they both cause serious diseases.

Where you live is a determining factor in how much toxicity these chlorines contain. For example, in Europe, cancer sufferers have higher amounts of polonium from chlorine, but they also have lower quantities of benzene and PCBs than those living elsewhere.

Dr. Clark says that all of the chlorines used have traces of polonium and cerium (a lathanide element), which are the first two components to forming cancer. The third component, which she says determines who will suffer from cancer, is whether it contains ferrocyanide or ferricyanide. She also discovered alpha radiation, antimony, arsenic, asbestos, azo dyes, barium, benzene, boron, and cadmium in the carcinogenic chlorine.

Are You Using Toxic Water?

Even if you are using mineral waters instead of commercially cleaned and supplied water, there are still risks to your safety and the proper function of your immune system that you need to be aware of.

During processing, mineral waters are introduced to toxins. Dr. Clark conducted examinations with a device she invented called the Syncrometer. Using this Syncrometer, a variety of water brands were tested, and it was found that immunosuppressants were present in many of them. In other words, even when the water itself is not dangerous, the bottling machines or the bottles themselves can be.

Water that is sold distilled can contain the same toxins as bottled mineral water and should also be avoided. As it is distilled, the water loses its toxins and passes through a charcoal filter that converts it into pure water containing no inorganic minerals. Because our bodies can't absorb these toxins, distilling water prevents them from depositing themselves on the walls of our intestines, arteries, joints, kidneys, etc.

Heavy metals are a big part of the problem when it comes to toxic foods, mostly because they can be so pervasive in our water and food supply. That said, according to Dr. Clark, there are several steps you can take to eliminate your exposure to heavy metals.

Your best bet is to distill your water yourself. If you must buy plastic packaging, Dr. Clark advises using an HDPE 2 plastic—mentioned above as the only safe form of plastic packaging—to avoid contamination. A glass container is also a safe and viable option.

You should also stay away from swordfish, tuna, bonito, shellfish, sea bass, eel, halibut, monkfish, salmon, sea bream, manta ray, and grouper. Dr. Clark advises sticking with varieties of fish that have a lower amount of mercury, like hake, whiting, blue whiting, sardine, herring, anchovy, and trout. These varieties give your body the much-needed nutrition without the high levels of heavy metal toxicity.

Antacids that contain aluminum hydroxide should be avoided, as should tobacco, which is a dangerous source of cadmium.

In the kitchen, dishes made out of clay and aluminum should be avoided, as should aluminum foil or tin. Relating to aluminum, pay attention to the packaging as well. Chocolate bars, chocolate eggs, and any food packaged in aluminum often can have unseen particles of aluminum attached to it.

Dr. Clark also cautions against vaccinations, as they are high in mercury and, though often recommended for various populations of people for different things (i.e., flu shots for the elderly, tetanus shots for farm workers), she says they are "frankly harmful."

Like all things, this is an area where we must strive for balance. Be aware of what is in the vaccinations, seek out all the necessary information, and come to an informed decision weighing the risks and benefits.

Put Your Body to Work

As you've seen from the frightening information above, fully avoiding toxins can be difficult—if not impossible—in today's world. The good news, however, is that our bodies contain several mechanisms to deal with certain levels of toxins in a healthy way. Namely, our white blood cells are the body's natural way of battling invaders.

But is conventional medicine right about the way white blood cells really work?

A familiar saying goes, "quality not quantity." That's true of our white blood cells. It's not how many white blood cells we have that's important. Rather, it's how well those cells are functioning that really matters when we look at health from the perspective of balance.

Just because our white blood cell count is within a normal range doesn't necessarily mean that the cells are functioning as they should in a natural state of homeostasis. For the many victims of disease, their white blood cell count isn't an issue, but the state of the cells is.

Traditional medicine has the ability to count our white blood cells, but not to evaluate their toxicity. This problem was remedied by Dr. Clark, who—as much discussed in this and previous chapters—is the author of several well-known books on the topic of self-health. Dr. Clark also used her Syncrometer device, discussed in one of the above sections, to see what she called "the five basic immunosuppressants" in her patients' white blood cells.

The "five basics" are not the only threatening toxins we consume, but according to Dr. Clark, they are the most relevant to our immune systems, as they are found in each and every person with degenerative diseases and infectious conditions. These immunosuppressants are PCBs (polychlorinated biphenyls), benzene, asbestos, azo dyes, and heavy metals, all of which we covered earlier in this chapter.

In a healthy state, our white blood cells can identify and react to invaders and disease. When they are "under the influence" of toxins, however, they are unable to perform primary functions like detecting and eliminating pathogens and toxins in the organs. The white blood cells are suddenly south polarized, rather than north polarized as they should be, thanks to the transportation of things like heavy metals for elimination.

Dr. Clark says that, because of this, when they can't eliminate toxins, white blood cells are not able to function, disrupting homeostasis in our bodies.

The obvious fix, then, is to detoxify the white blood cells so that our immune systems can work properly. Our white blood cells need to be prepared to release toxins into the bladder and excrete them through urine. In order to do this, Dr. Clark says we need to get our immune system strong so that it can eliminate any toxins that enter the body altogether.

To go up against pathogens and toxins, our white blood cells need one important thing from us: non-toxic nourishment, a critical part of creating homeostasis in our diet.

Detoxify Your Diet

Small and simple changes can have a significant effect on your body's ability to rid itself of toxins and return to a state of homeostasis. The foods you eat and the water you drink are two simple dietary needs you can control with minimal effort and maximum effect.

In order to cleanse our bodies of toxins, we need to have white blood cells that are doing their job for us. Eliminating heavy metals from our lives and making educated choices when it comes to the food we eat and the water we use will help our bodies complete their natural toxin-fighting duties, restoring balance and returning us to the Wellness Model of Health™.

But toxic foods aren't the only things we need to be on the lookout for when it comes to our diets. Next, I'll show you how you may be consuming mold without knowing it, and how you can eliminate it from your food intake to improve your health.

The Truth about Mold

While it is easy to grasp the concept of toxins in our food and water, you may be less aware of another factor in your environment that can have serious repercussions for your health and wellness: molds.

Molds are a form of fungus, usually microscopic, that live and reproduce on organic matter such as plants or animals. While the word "mold" tends to have a negative connotation, it actually describes a diverse group of organisms, some beneficial and some harmful.

Most of us are aware that mold plays a critical role in our ecosystem. When living things die, mold sets in and makes them biodegradable. Without it, our land and oceans would be bursting with all of the dead plants and animals from years gone by. Mold works in a miraculous way to get rid of filth.

Mold consumption impacts the diet aspect of the Complete Healing Formula™. That's not to say that all molds are bad for you. Some of them are actually beneficial. Many delicious and healthy cheeses owe their existence to healthy molds. The species *Penicillium roqueforti* is the key mold that gives Gorgonzola, Stilton, and the aptly named Roquefort cheeses their distinct flavors and appearances. Beyond these three, many other cheeses likewise require other safe, edible kinds of molds in the mix to craft their appealing flavors.

But not all molds are beneficial to your dietary balance. On the contrary, we also encounter several toxic and dangerous forms of mold in our daily lives. Your food pantry, your bread, your fruit basket, the rind of your orange, and the walls of your kitchen themselves are just a few places where these toxic molds can grow—with dangerous and sometimes even life-threatening repercussions for your health.

Estimates suggest that there are anywhere from tens of thousands to hundreds of thousands of mold species. Covering them all in this chapter is simply impossible. Fortunately, it's also unnecessary. The most valuable things to understand are why certain molds are dangerous and how you can identify them.

Some molds are visible; others are invisible. Some are helpful; others are extremely dangerous. Regardless of the mold, however, most require certain conditions to spread and thrive. Once you know those conditions, you can avoid them and work toward greater balance in your diet.

The next few pages will explain how molds form, cover the different types of molds that can adversely affect your health, and show you how to manage mold consumption in your diet.

The Dangers of Mold

What are molds, how do they spread, and why are they harmful to our overall health?

Molds are composed of pervasive roots—specifically, from stalks rising out of those roots that are capped off with spores. We can see these spores with the naked eye. The spores are what give molds their individual appearances and colors, and they are also the source of the molds' dangerous effects.

Mold spores spread through the environment through the air. Certain molds, such as those found in some buildings, give off spores that cause allergic reactions and respiratory problems. The presence of mold in a home is rightly a cause for grave concern. Until the molds are eliminated, and their spores cleared from the atmosphere, the environment is toxic.

Many molds have a more pervasive and dangerous effect on our health than simple allergies. Several types of molds produce "mycotoxins," which, as their name suggests, are extremely toxic. Worse, many molds have extremely intricate root systems, which allow mycotoxins to penetrate far deeper into a substance than the visible spores lead us to believe.

Each grain, fruit, tea and coffee plant, herb, and vegetable has its molds— and, odds are, you're eating them.

Aflatoxin

Aflatoxin is one of the more pervasive and toxic molds out there. This is no surprise given the conditions in which it thrives best. Aflatoxin is found primarily on corn and peanuts, both of which are staples of the modern American diet.

This mold is recognized by the USDA as a cancer-causing poison. So it comes as no surprise that Dr. Hulda Clark's research uncovered aflatoxin in virtually all of her cancer patients. Aflatoxin also appeared in all of Dr. Clark's cases of hepatitis and cirrhosis. This mold attacks the body's immune system, leaving the gates of our defenses wide open to pathogens.

Aflatoxin is not easily cleared from the body because it weakens and kills portions of the liver—the organ that is meant to detoxify our systems. Large doses or continued exposure to this mold will harm your health through its detrimental effects on the liver. That said, it can take weeks for aflatoxin's effects to be realized, and it is both tasteless and scentless. So how can you know if your food is moldy?

In addition to thriving on corn and peanuts, aflatoxin is also found in your cereal, bread, pasta, nuts, maple syrup, orange juice, and other foods. The good news is that it is not found in dairy, fresh-washed produce, or water. Goods produced in bakeries that are left open to air also don't contain aflatoxin, and the same is true for products made with carefully screened, deseeded wheat.

In short, given the common American diet, the possibility that you are consuming foods riddled with aflatoxin is very likely unless you take the proper steps to avoid this moldy invader. Dr. Clark advises preparing your own food, testing the foods you can't prepare yourself, treating foods for molds whenever you can, and getting rid of the rest of it.

One of the most important things to understand is that you can't kill molds through the basic heating or reheating of food. Foods containing aflatoxin must be boiled for several minutes—at a temperature much higher than the boiling point—or else be baked at an even higher temperature in order to kill this mold. So if your food can't be heated to an elevated temperature, this method will not kill the aflatoxin.

Some industrial research journals suggest treating food ingredients with hydrogen peroxide or metabisulfite, a reducing agent. While the introduction of these chemicals may kill the mold, however, that's not their only effect. They also damage the nutritional value of your food—not to mention its flavor.

The only natural way to ensure that your food isn't infested with aflatoxin, as Dr. Clark suggests, is through the use of vitamin C. Be advised that you should use whole-food vitamin C for this, not ascorbic acid. Ascorbic acid is not true vitamin C, but rather a chemical compound, as I will discuss later in this book. Only real vitamin C will have the purifying effect on your food that Dr. Clark identifies.

When baking your own bread, Dr. Clark advises adding a bit of vitamin C to the dough to keep it free of mold for a longer time. In both powdered and liquid forms, vitamin C is an easy way to quickly ensure the safety of your food. Still, be sure to consume the bread quickly, or slice and freeze it to prevent the resurgence of the aflatoxin.

Purchasing commercially available bread is dangerous, since vitamin C can't be added before baking, and you can't be sure how long the bread has been sitting on the shelves in a store or bakery since it was made.

Other foods are also easy to treat with vitamin C. Rice and pasta can be cleansed of aflatoxin simply be adding vitamin C during or immediately after cooking. Vinegar can be detoxified as well simply by adding some vitamin C before refrigerating it. You can even rid honey of mold if you heat it slightly and add a few tablespoons of vitamin C to the container.

Some foods, like nuts, need a slightly different treatment. Simply sprinkling vitamin C on nuts or corn will not remove the aflatoxin from these foods because they have already been penetrated by molds. Nuts have to be washed and covered with water that has been mixed with vitamin C powder. After five minutes, the vitamin C has detoxed the nuts and they can be dried in the oven using low heat.

Interestingly, many cultures traditionally treat corn in a way that naturally clears it of aflatoxin. The process that these cultures use is called "nixtamalization," which involves soaking and cooking corn in a limewater solution. This alkalizes the corn, and the presence of vitamin C in the limewater rids it of aflatoxin.

Avoid the harmful effects of aflatoxin by steering clear of the common foods where this mold appears whenever you can, to ensure it doesn't enter your system. However, keep in mind that, because the foods on which aflatoxin thrives are so common, a preventative treatment cleanse is also necessary to avoid ingesting this cancer-causing organism. I'll talk more about cleanses in chapter 15.

Zearalenone

Zearalenone, or "zear" is another common and dangerous mold to avoid. Like its cousin aflatoxin, zear is often found in commercial cereal grains and processed foods such as popcorn, corn chips, and brown rice.

Zear can lower your immunity, just as aflatoxin does. It furthermore keeps your body from being able to detoxify benzene, which Dr. Clark says is common in AIDS sufferers. In addition, this mold is linked with estrogen-dependent diseases, including breast cancer.

Another mycotoxin, zear is an anabolic and estrogenic metabolite. The mold appears as extra estrogen in animals' bodies. Many animal studies have shown this mold to have negative impacts on reproductive health, such as infertility and in-utero death.

But such negative effects are not limited to animals. Even beyond breast cancer, Dr. Clark found in her research that zear speeds up the maturing process in females, and could cause PMS, ovarian cysts, and infertility. In males, even small amounts of zear ingested daily could dramatically affect maturation. Whether the toxin stimulates additional estrogen to develop or functions just like estrogen is not yet clear.

High heat is not effective when it comes to purging foods of zear. If your immunity is compromised or you experience any of the other effects noted above, Dr. Clark advises going off moldy food suspects that may contain zear right away.

Ergot

Ergot is a mold whose effects are unusual and felt very fast. It is immune to heat and highly toxic to children. At any age, however, erratic behavior can be a consequence of ingesting ergot. Irrational thoughts, surreal ideas, and unusual emotions are significant red flags. Those who are commonly sick may also be experiencing high levels of this toxin. According to Dr. Clark, the effects of ergot also include paranoia, hearing voices, and even seizures.

If you notice any of these erratic behaviors in yourself or someone you are close to, it would be a good idea to make dietary changes to reduce your intake of ergot.

For example, erratic behavior in children is often written off as allergies, when in truth ergot toxicity could be to blame. If you find your child behaving like "Jekyll and Hyde," Dr. Clark suggests eliminating cold cereals, nuts and nut butters, store-bought baked goods, soy, honey, and syrups for three weeks. Replace those foods with hot cereals, home-baked goods, potatoes, and honey with added vitamin C.

Because alcohol together with ergot is more toxic than each is on its own, alcohol heightens the negative effects of ergot. It appears that alcohol also drives ergot deeper into the tissues. Dr. Clark has found ergot and aflatoxin in beer and wine, and suggests that perhaps some inebriated behaviors are the result of this mold and alcohol combination.

If you intend to consume foods that may contain ergot, Dr. Clark notes that you can detoxify this dangerous mold easily in about ten minutes using Vitamin C. She also notes that honey should be detoxified right away before consumption.

Other Molds to Avoid

Aflatoxin, zearalenone, and ergot are only a few of the toxic molds we need to reduce or eliminate in our diets. There are several other molds to be aware of as well.

Cytochalasin B

Cytochalasin B, or "cyto B," is another fungus that lowers immunity, which it does by impeding cell division. For example, portions of the liver that are dead are unable to regenerate as they normally would in the event of a toxic encounter. Cyto B it is found mainly in pasta.

Kojic Acid

Kojic acid prevents the body from being able to detoxify wood alcohol, which results in damage to the pancreas, pancreatic fluke infestation, and even diabetes. Dr. Clark advises against eating potato skins and points out that this mold is also found in regular coffee.

T-2 Toxin

Dr. Clark has found T-2 toxin in every case of high blood pressure and kidney disease. She notes that it is found in dried peas and beans, but that this dangerous mold can be detoxified by adding vitamin C to the soaking water for these foods for five minutes. She adds that you should discard the imperfect peas and beans first, as an extra safety measure.

Sorghum Molds

Sorghum molds are found in sorghum and millet. Elderly people are more susceptible to these mold toxins, which cause hemorrhaging and appetite loss, and make it hard to swallow. Dr. Clark advises against buying sorghum syrup, and says that you should rinse millet in water with vitamin C or add vitamin C to the water before cooking.

Patulin

Patulin is the major fruit mold toxin. It is dangerous because the mold that produces it can grow in patches in your intestine. According to Dr. Clark, E. coli and shigella can permeate the colon wall and begin to invade your body, spreading to areas of injury and tumor sites.

Patulin is found in many common fruits when they are bruised. Those with bowel disease or cancer should not consume fresh fruit besides bananas and lemons for a few weeks. After that, all fruit should be carefully inspected for bruising, and Dr. Clark warns to be thorough in the inspection: even a single soft grape can reinfect you.

Mold and Your Diet

The following are foods Dr. Clark says should be carefully considered prior to consumption:

- Crackers: Children should not be fed crackers ever as they are notoriously moldy. Make your own treats in the oven.

- Dried fruits: These are highly moldy and should be soaked in vitamin C water and refrigerated or frozen. Overripe fruit should not be baked or preserved.

- Peanut butter: Nut butters bought in a store can't be detoxified, so you should make your own.

- Tea: Tea sold in bags is very moldy, so it is better to buy tea in bulk. Store tea in the double plastic bag it comes in, which will also prevent antiseptics in the bag itself. When using fresh herbs, only half as much is required to make tea, which should be done using a sterile bamboo strainer.

- Maple syrup: Pure maple syrup contains aflatoxin and other molds that you can often see. The aflatoxin can be removed with vitamin C, but the other molds need to be exposed to high heat too. You can bring the syrup to a near boil in its original jar without the lid and then refrigerate.

- Hot cereal: It is easy to spot the mold here and remove all of the dark shriveled pieces. By adding salt and honey while cooking, you can detoxify your hot cereal grains further. Grains shouldn't sit in your cupboard for more than six months, and should not be refrigerated (only frozen) if not kept in the cupboard.

Against the Grains

According to Dr. Clark, our grain consumption should be very limited. Many molds in pastas, breads, and cold cereals can't be seen or smelled. Potatoes are a preferable option, as you eat them just the way they were harvested. When grains are processed, it opens them to a variety of molds. Potatoes should be scrubbed prior to eating, and all eyes should be removed.

Coexisting with Mold

Mold could be called a necessary evil. While it is vital to the balance of the environment, if not carefully monitored, it can make us very sick in a variety of ways. It is not complicated to co-exist with mold, but it does require diligence on our parts to make sure that what we put into our bodies is as safe as it can be.

Keep in mind that you don't have to go to extremes with this all at once. The first step is knowledge and awareness. Once you have that, you can start taking small steps to reduce your exposure to molds, then build on it over time. This is only one part of the bigger picture when it comes to managing excesses, deficiencies, and stagnations in your diet.

Now you're aware of the serious threats that toxic and moldy foods pose to our dietary balance, and how they can undermine the Wellness Model of Health™. But there is one more culprit when it comes to sabotaging health through diet: inflammatory foods. The next chapter will take you through everything you need to know about these foods, and show you how you can eliminate them from your diet to promote greater wellness.

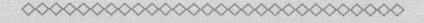

Chapter Review

- Toxic foods harm our white blood cells and weaken our immune systems.

- Five common immunosuppressants you should try to avoid most in foods are: polychlorinated biphenyls (PCBs), benzene, asbestos, azo dyes, and heavy metals.

- Molds are a form of fungus, usually microscopic, that live and reproduce on organic matter such as plants or animals.

- Some forms of mold are toxic and dangerous, and can be found in common foods we eat.

- Mold spores spread through the environment through the air.

- Some foods that commonly contain mold include: crackers, dried fruits, peanut butter, tea, maple syrup, and hot cereal, as well as pastas, breads, cold cereals, grains, and potatoes.

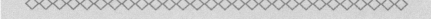

Recommended Resources

ElectroCleanse

Developed by the Dr. Clark Research Association, the ElectroCleanse is a powerful tool that can aid you in the recovery of many major medical disorders. Find out more at www.losethebackpain.com/productreviews/electrocleanse.html.

Dr. Clark Research Association

You can learn more about the tools available to clear toxins from your system from the Dr. Clark Research Association at www.drclark.com.

Clark Therapy by Ignacio Chamorro Balda

You can get even more information about the tools and methods that have arisen from Dr. Clark's work in the book *Clark Therapy* by Ignacio Chamorro Balda.

CHAPTER 12:

Everyday Foods that Fan the Flames of Inflammation

Inflammation Station

I spent a lot of time in the last chapter giving you the rundown of what dangerous things may be coming along with your food. But if you're like most people, some of the foods you eat may be harmful for your health in and of themselves.

In today's fad diet world, it's probably no surprise to hear that what you eat is important to creating homeostasis in the Wellness Model of Health™. The food you consume has far more of an impact on you than just the weight it may add to your frame. Beyond the obvious, certain foods can create an excess of inflammation within the body, triggering pain and ill-health.

The impact of inflammation on the body is enormous. For example, inflammation in joints causes stiffness and pain. Inflammation in the back and muscles results in trigger points. Arterial inflammation is associated with heart disease, and fascia-related inflammation is linked strongly to fibromyalgia. In fact, multiple studies have proven that inflammation is connected to nearly every major disease we suffer from today. And it starts with the food you eat every single day—the third cornerstone of the Complete Healing Formula™, your diet.

By now, you know that diet has an impact on our physical and mental well-being. No matter what kind of pain or illness you're suffering from, you're going to make your whole situation and state of homeostasis better by improving your diet. There are specific conditions that many people suffer from—like chronic joint pain—that can be alleviated by following simple dietary guidelines.

An obvious example, as Dr. Mark Wiley cites in his book, *Arthritis Reversed,* is that if you are carrying around excess weight, it places a compressive load on your joints that is three times the actual weight. That means for every fifteen pounds you are overweight, your hips and knees are under stress to move a forty-five-pound load. If you are thirty to forty pounds or more overweight, the effects can be staggering.

Changing the way you eat to reduce your level of chronic inflammation will most likely lead to weight loss, which will in turn result in the relief of excess pressure on your body. And this is only one superficial way that inflammation impacts our larger health ecosystem.

In addition to eating well, there are specific foods you can avoid and others you can consume to preserve and improve your body's defense against inflammation, your natural state of homeostasis, and consequently, your health conditions.

This chapter will review how food causes pain and inflammation, which foods affect inflammation, and how you can ease pain and discomfort with a diet of healthy whole foods.

How Food Causes Pain and Inflammation

When it comes to pain and inflammation, the food you consume plays a key role. Food is a critical piece of the puzzle when it comes to controlling energy-draining health symptoms.

Unfortunately, the typical American diet consists of excess fat, tons of sugar, loads of factory-farmed red meat, and a frightening amount of processed foods. Is it any wonder there are so many people suffering from chronic pain and illness? These foods cause inflammation, block the bowels, drain the immune system, and deplete the blood of dense nutrients.

"Bad" Foods

When it comes to pain and illness, several categories of food should be avoided, including nightshades, dairy-based products, and high-fructose corn syrup. Dr. Wiley covers a number of these in his book.

Excess nightshade fruits and vegetables are particularly troublesome for those suffering from conditions like chronic joint pain. This family of food includes white potatoes, eggplant, sweet and hot peppers, tomatoes, tomatillos, tamarillos, pepinos, pimentos, goji berries, ground cherries, Cape gooseberries, garden huckleberries, and paprika.

These foods can cause calcification, bone spurs, and inflammation. Such side effects are harmful to those suffering pain and illness because they amplify the existing inflammation and joint problems rather than alleviating them. In cases of people who are sensitive or allergic to nightshades, they can even cause nerve damage, muscle tremors, and impeded digestion.

Excess dairy products are also troublesome for those suffering from chronic ailments. They are often high in cholesterol and saturated fat, and can contribute to obesity. And as we learned, being overweight by even fifteen pounds can have disastrous effects on arthritic joints. But the problem with dairy goes a lot deeper than weight issues.

Products like milk, yogurt, ice cream, cheese, cottage cheese, and various sauces can contribute to an increase in phlegm-rheum. Phlegm-rheum is a classification of thick, sticky fluids in the body that include mucus. These thick and sticky fluids pool around joints and collect toxins and bacteria, and become either damp or hot, depending on other factors. This increases inflammation, swelling, bone degeneration, loss of range of motion, and pain.

The sweetener known as high-fructose corn syrup (HFC) has been called the main culprit in the rise in youth obesity in the United States, and obesity is one of the key risks for chronic health issues. High-fructose corn syrup is corn syrup that has undergone enzymatic processing to convert its glucose into fructose. This fructose has then been mixed with regular corn syrup, which is 100 percent glucose, and the result is a sweet liquid known as high-fructose.

This liquid is the sweetener found in just about every cold beverage in your local convenience store, including iced tea, sodas, and energy drinks. Not only that, but it is also found in so-called healthy foods like tomato soup and yogurt, as well as less healthful items such as salad dressings and cookies.

The FDA did a thirty-year study and found a correlation between HFC and obesity, stating that it is worse for your health than plain sugar—which isn't good for those with pain and inflammation either. Worst of all, even as the public begins to awaken to the dangers of HFC, the food industry is now peddling equally dangerous chemical sugar substitutes and all the additional toxins that come with them.

Excess processed or refined grains are also to be avoided. These are found in flour, cereals, breads, baked goods, and snack foods. Usually they're listed as "enriched" flour or anything other than "whole" grains. In essence, refined grains have been broken down for you, so your body doesn't have to do the work.

Since the grain then breaks down too quickly in the body and the intestines, it releases hormones that promote inflammation. Even eating "whole" grains can still be problematic for many people. Not only are those whole grains still processed, but many grains—especially wheat—trigger inflammatory responses in the body.

Acidic Foods

Other foods that negatively affect our health include those that are acidic. As strange as it may sound, your body, its fluids, and your blood can become excessively acidic. Just as acidic fruits like lemons can "eat" the enamel off your teeth, and acid can corrode a battery casing, your body can become overly acidic when your natural pH is off kilter.

Even the conventional medical community agrees that the human body was not designed to withstand chronic acidic states. When the body is off-kilter long enough, out of its natural state of homeostasis, it starts to break down.

Signs and symptoms of an excessively acidic body can be seen and/or felt externally, with the onset of headaches, body pain, and skin rashes. In the acidic range, the immune system is compromised, leading to easily contracted sinus infections, allergies, colds, and the flu, and placing you at risk for progressing autoimmune diseases and rheumatoid arthritis.

Moreover, an excessively acidic interior environment can lead to muscle contraction that can restrict the free flow of blood and inhibit the exchange of nutrients and waste products from muscle cells. This can cause soreness, cramping, fatigue, degenerative cellular diseases, and even cellular death. Dr. Wiley offers a pH balance guide in his book, reproduced here.

Chart 12.1: pH Balance Guide

Acid	0	Battery Acid
	1	Stomach Acid
	2	Lemon Juice, Vinegar
	3	Orange Juice, Soda
	4	Tomato Juice, Beer
	5	Black Coffee
	6	Saliva, Cow's Milk
Neutral	7	Pure Water
Alkaline	8	Sea Water
	9	Baking Soda
	10	Antacid
	11	Ammonia
	12	Soapy Water
	13	Bleach, Oven Cleaner
	14	Drain Cleaner

Chronic pain is related to pH imbalance and the accumulation of acid deposits in the joints of the neck, hips, wrists, and hands. It is this accumulated acid that damages cartilage. When the cells that produce lubricating synovial fluids and bursa fluids are acidic, this condition causes a dryness that irritates and swells the joints. When uric acid builds up, it tends to deposit in the form of crystals that can feel like broken glass in the feet, hands, knees, and back.

Thankfully, you don't have to worry about this when your body is kept within the alkaline range of 7.0 - 7.4. In fact, while in this range it is impossible for disease to sustain itself, because the immune system is strong and the acidic environment necessary for diseases like cancer, gout, and arthritis no longer exists. Chart 12.1 will help you see just how the foods you eat and the beverages you drink contribute to an unhealthy internal environment.

Acidity and Stress

An imbalanced pH or acid/alkaline interior environment is one of the hidden causes of disease and one of the states that makes our existing health symptoms worse.

So how does the body become too acidic (and thus, unhealthy) and place you at risk for negative health symptoms? Well, excess stress is a big one.

As I discussed in chapter 2, stress, or the effects of being in the "fight or flight" response for too long a period of time, releases stress hormones into the body, flooding the blood stream with protective chemicals. These chemicals, like cortisol, were necessary during the times of our ancestors who had to run for their lives from wild beasts or rival tribes.

These days, this stress response is caused by different types of stressors, like emotional upset, physically demanding work, and overwhelming psychological issues that we deal with at home and at work. There are too many of these happening throughout the day. It is no wonder we are under chronic states of stress, are not well, and are in a constant acidic state.

Our modern diet is also a huge contributor to our chronic acidic interior environment. When food reaches your digestive tract, it is broken down and either leaves an alkaline or an acidic residue behind. If you eat foods that are organic, whole, and fresh, and drink plenty of pure water, the body can easily maintain an alkaline state.

However, consuming excess sugar, refined grains, preservatives, pesticides, dairy products (like cow's milk, cheese, yogurt, and ice cream), red meat, chocolate, coffee, soda and alcohol turns the body acidic. One of the main effects of a poor diet is inflammation, which is also the main symptom of chronic pain and illness.

pH is a measure of the potential hydrogen or residue a food leaves behind, as being either alkaline or acidic. And this is not directly related to the acidic nature of a food before it is digested. Lemons, for example, are highly acidic. If you squeeze the juice of a lemon on an open wound, it will burn. However, when ingested and digested, lemon is very alkalizing for the body, and lemon juice can help reduce acidic levels. A diet that is low in acidic foods and packed full of nutrient-dense alkalizing foods will make you healthier, while also reducing the symptoms of your chronic pain or illness.

If you have pain or chronic disease, you more than likely have a predisposition to infection, and it is likely that a pH imbalance is present in your body. To be sure, you can purchase pH testing strips or rolls in your local drug store.

These are thin paper items that gauge your pH level when dipped either into your saliva or urine stream, first thing in the morning before anything is eaten or drunk. You should strive to have your pH in in the alkaline range, and if you aren't at that level, you should try to move closer to it each day.

Good Foods

Now for the good news. There are plenty of foods that you can add to your daily diet to make you strong and keep you in homeostatic balance. A diet high in fiber and whole foods, low in preservatives and unhealthy fat, and infused with blood-invigorating aromatic spices can help reduce pain and inflammation.

It is essential to any healthful diet that you consume as many fresh, organic, whole foods as possible. Eating foods in or close to their original state is one of the keys to being healthy, preventing self-induced diet-based inflammation, and reducing the inflammation you are experiencing as a result of your pain or illness.

Dr. Wiley's book, *Arthritis Reversed*, gives a concise list of the best foods known to prevent and help reduce inflammation and pain. These should be eaten throughout the day as part of balanced wholesome meals.

- Wild fish (example: Alaskan salmon)
- Fresh whole fruits
- Bright colored vegetables (except nightshades)

- Green and white tea
- Purified and distilled water
- Healthy oils (coconut, olive, flax, hemp, safflower, hazelnut)
- Beef and poultry that is certified organic, grass fed, soy free, and free range
- Nuts, legumes, and seeds
- Dark green leafy vegetables
- Organic oatmeal (regular, not instant)
- Aromatic spices (turmeric, ginger, cloves, garlic, onion, coriander, and ground mustard seed)

I want to stress the importance of making sure your meat comes from animals that are grass fed, soy free, free range, and certified organic. It is a sad truth that a lot of the meat that is commercially available today comes from sick animals, who are kept in awful, unhealthy, and cruel conditions.

These animals are usually stuffed and packed into barns so tightly they can barely move and they get little to no natural light. They are also often given growth hormones and overfed with foods they wouldn't eat normally, like corn for cows and, in some cases, even dead, sick animals. These conditions obviously make the animals sick, and then they need antibiotics. At the end of this cycle, the unhealthy, antibiotic-ridden, hormone-laced meat from a sick animal finds its way into our bodies. That's why it's so important to choose your meat with care.

As you can see, a diet high in whole foods and low in preservatives and unhealthy fat is an essential part of any pain and illness relief plan. Not only do the above-listed foods actually work to reduce pain and inflammation, but they also support proper nerve function, and muscle and bone health.

Remember, the acid/alkaline or pH level of your body (which can cause or prevent inflammation), is related to the foods you consume. Using the chart reproduced from Dr. Wiley's *Arthritis Reversed* below, see how what you consume on a daily or monthly basis may be contributing to the worsening of your chronic health condition.

Chart 12.2: pH Spectrum

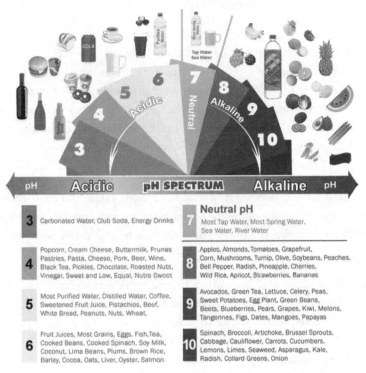

3	Carbonated Water, Club Soda, Energy Drinks	**7**	**Neutral pH** Most Tap Water, Most Spring Water, Sea Water, River Water
4	Popcorn, Cream Cheese, Buttermilk, Prunes Pastries, Pasta, Cheese, Pork, Beer, Wine, Black Tea, Pickles, Chocolate, Roasted Nuts, Vinegar, Sweet and Low, Equal, Nutra Sweet	**8**	Apples, Almonds, Tomatoes, Grapefruit, Corn, Mushrooms, Turnip, Olive, Soybeans, Peaches, Bell Pepper, Radish, Pineapple, Cherries, Wild Rice, Apricot, Strawberries, Bananas
5	Most Purified Water, Distilled Water, Coffee, Sweetened Fruit Juice, Pistachios, Beef, White Bread, Peanuts, Nuts, Wheat,	**9**	Avocados, Green Tea, Lettuce, Celery, Peas, Sweet Potatoes, Egg Plant, Green Beans, Beets, Blueberries, Pears, Grapes, Kiwi, Melons, Tangerines, Figs, Dates, Mangoes, Papayas
6	Fruit Juices, Most Grains, Eggs, Fish, Tea, Cooked Beans, Cooked Spinach, Soy Milk, Coconut, Lima Beans, Plums, Brown Rice, Barley, Cocoa, Oats, Liver, Oyster, Salmon	**10**	Spinach, Broccoli, Artichoke, Brussel Sprouts, Cabbage, Cauliflower, Carrots, Cucumbers, Lemons, Limes, Seaweed, Asparagus, Kale, Radish, Collard Greens, Onion

Credit: mindbodygreen.com http://www.mindbodygreen.com/0-5165/Alkaline-Acidic-Foods-Chart-The-pH-Spectrum.html

Green Tea

Dr. Wiley did a significant amount of research on green tea. He found that green tea, like all true tea, comes from the leaves of the Camellia Sinensis tree, and 90 percent of the world's tea supply is produced in China. What makes green tea so powerful is a chemical compound called polyphenol, which occurs naturally in plants and works as an antioxidant.

Polyphenols work to protect the body from the oxidative stress that causes diseases. Specifically, the polyphenol Epigallocatechin gallate (EGCG) is an extremely powerful antioxidant. In fact, EGCG antioxidant activity is more powerful than the antioxidants found in vitamins C and E.

After fifteen years of working with green tea in his cancer research, Dr. Hasan Mukhtar started looking at the possible benefits this drink could have for people with rheumatoid arthritis. Realizing that both disorders were inflammatory in nature, his team began testing to see if green tea would have the same healing effect on rheumatoid arthritis as it does on cancer and cardiovascular disease.

His first paper, "Prevention of Collagen-Induced Arthritis in Mice by a Polyphenolic Fraction of Green Tea," was presented to the National Academy of Sciences in April 2005. The results were astounding. Out of the eighteen mice that were given green tea extract, ten never developed any arthritic symptoms. What's more, symptoms in the remaining eight showed that they developed a much milder form of arthritis. The amount given was the equivalent of drinking just four cups of green tea a day!

Lead author of the paper, Dr. Tariq M. Haqqi said, "Taken together, our studies suggest that a polyphenolic fraction from green tea that is rich in antioxidants may be useful in the prevention and onset and severity of arthritis."

Three independent and controlled experiments were conducted. Using a widely accepted animal model that is very similar to rheumatoid arthritis, the mice were injected with collagen to induce arthritis. Two groups were studied for forty days, while a third was examined for eighty-five days to verify that the green tea did not simply delay the onset of the disease.

Green tea, unlike the more widely used black version, is not fermented. Instead of crushing the tea leaves, thereby removing the polyphenols, green tea is first dried, and then heated. One teaspoon steeped in hot (not boiling) water contains anywhere from 100 to 200mg of EGCG. Milk should not be added, as it negates the tea's beneficial properties. According to this study and others that were done for other diseases, two to four cups a day is usually recommended.

Human trials are currently being developed. In the meantime, however,.Drs. Mukhtar and Haqqi both strongly encourage people to start drinking green tea. Nobody has shown any form of toxicity associated with tea, and with the tremendous amount of data showing its many beneficial qualities, it is a wise and wholesome preventive measure.

Mushrooms

Mushrooms should also be a part of your daily diet, as they are full of nutrients and are power immune boosters.

There are many reasons that mushrooms are so powerful and essential to our health. They are an excellent dietary staple and health booster, containing nine of the essential amino acids our bodies need, along with 30 percent of the high-quality proteins we require. Plus, with virtually no unsaturated fat, they include more minerals than most meat and vegetables.

Even more important than their nutritional content, mushrooms are rich in enzymes that are critical to reducing inflammation throughout the body. For this reason, mushrooms are known to be useful in alleviating rheumatoid arthritis symptoms, hypertension and heart disease, diabetes, and even some cancers.

With so much going for them, and all their amazing health benefits, what's not to love? So go ahead and give mushrooms a big welcome in your home. Add them to your meals where you can. You will feel a whole lot better because of it.

Turmeric

In cultures that are thousands of years old, such as in India, there are deep traditions of cooking daily meals with medicinal roots and herbs. These herbs act as preventive measures for sustaining good health, and prevention is the cornerstone of India's traditional Ayurvedic medicine. Turmeric is one such medicinal root that has made its way into a vast number of Indian recipes.

Aside from your standard chicken or goat curries, there is a whole list of Indian dishes that contain flavorful thermogenic ingredients like cardamom, coriander, ginger, cloves, and turmeric. Not only are these recipes tasty, the ones containing turmeric are especially healthful because of one of its components, called curcumin.

Research conducted by Sarker et al. notes the powerful anti-inflammatory, anti-tumor, and antioxidant properties of curcumin. Moreover, the US National Library of Medicine and the National Institutes of Health say: "Laboratory and animal research has demonstrated anti-inflammatory, antioxidant, and anti-cancer properties of turmeric and its constituent curcumin."

Unlike aspirin or ibuprofen, turmeric's curcumin reduces inflammation naturally, without damaging the liver or kidneys. It has been found especially helpful in treating conditions like arthritis, sports injuries, irritable bowel syndrome, Crohn's disease, tendonitis, and various autoimmune diseases. Some research even suggests that curcumin may also help those suffering asthma, inflammatory bowel disease, and yes, even cancer.

Since curcumin is an anti-inflammatory as well as an antioxidant, it is used for treating arthritis, wounds, digestive disorders, liver issues, and in the prevention of cancer. It also helps reduce the side effects of chemotherapy. Statistics show that Asian children experience less incidence of leukemia than their Western counterparts, and a diet rich in turmeric may be the reason why.

With no negative effects, there's no reason not to include more turmeric in your diet. You can try to eat more Indian and Malaysian food or buy the ground powder and use it in your own cooking. Since the flavor can be strong, some people prefer to purchase a high-quality curcumin supplement. In any case, make turmeric and curcumin part of your diet and start reducing your body's inflammation.

Inflammation Free

Being aware of what you're eating and how it affects your body. Think about this in the larger context of the Wellness Model of Health™. This is the first step toward becoming free of inflammation. By tweaking your diet to avoid certain foods and adding some new ones, you can live an overall healthier and happier life.

And good food isn't the only tool you have at your disposal when it comes to building better wellness. In the next chapter, I'll talk about the power of hydration and show you how simple water has the power to change your life.

Chapter Review

- Inflammation is associated with nearly every major disease we suffer from today.

- The typical American diet is filled with foods that cause inflammation.

- Acidic foods are another cause of inflammation. Stress can cause additional acidity in the body.

- A diet high in fiber and whole foods, low in preservatives and unhealthy fat, and infused with blood-invigorating aromatic spices can help reduce pain and inflammation.

- Green tea, mushrooms, and turmeric are extra-strong foods for battling inflammation.

Recommended Resources

Arthritis Reversed by Dr. Mark Wiley

You can get a detailed list of the best and worst foods for inflammation in Dr. Mark Wiley's book, *Arthritis Reversed* at www.arthritisbookfree.com.

CHAPTER 13:

Are Your Insides Like a Dried-Out Sponge?

Raise a Glass to Your Health

Here's a question that a lot of people ask me: Is water really that important?

Yes, it really is. For those suffering from chronic pain and illness, water is an absolutely critical element on the journey back optimal wellness.

Getting enough water every day is essential to the diet aspect of the Complete Healing Formula™, and it is vital to your health and well-being. In fact, one of the first things you can do at home when you're not feeling well is to take a look at how much water you've consumed so far that day. As a chronically dehydrated society, we'd all do well to "drink to our health."

Since water makes up roughly 75 percent of the human body (and 85 percent of the brain), it makes sense that no tissue, organ, or gland can function properly without ample supply of this natural fluid. Just as we use water to douse the flames of a house fire, we can use it to help cool our body's inflammation. Water is the primary tool for cleaning stains and dirt from our homes, and it is critical for washing toxins from our bodies as well.

To put it simply: we humans would cease to exist without the water. And it's no wonder that hydration plays such a major role in creating homeostasis in the Wellness Model of Health™.

This chapter will discuss why hydration is important for our bodies, how it relates to pain, and how you can hydrate properly.

Why Hydration Is Important

When talking about diet, water often is ignored. Yet it should be the first item on the list.

Water is the lifeblood of our existence, second only to air. Without it, we wouldn't survive much longer than three or so days. It cleans out toxins, hydrates tissues and organs, regulates body temperature, and supplies oxygen, which is involved in nearly all chemical processes in the body.

The mere consumption of water can help restore the body to its natural state of homeostasis (balance) by clearing toxins, cleansing the colon, flushing the liver and kidneys, and emptying the bowels.

As the water content of our tissues falls to a certain point because of dehydration (deficiency), the bi-layer membranes that surround cells contract, forming a barrier that prevents further water loss. This self-preservation tactic also obstructs the free movement of molecules, so metabolism and elimination are limited.

Once the cells have constricted themselves to preserve water, our metabolism slows and waste products in and around the cells are not eliminated, creating a stagnation of toxins in the blood. This toxic build-up in the blood often manifests as chemically-induced headaches, fibromyalgia, and the pain and inflammation associated with arthritis.

Pain or discomfort is usually the body's warning sign to drink more water before more serious problems begin to spread. In other words, a deficiency of water causes the body's natural cleaning processes to slow, building up toxins that create all sorts of illnesses and pain, which can get out of control if we chronically ignore them.

Most of us can easily understand why water is necessary to keep our blood cleansing processes flowing smoothly. The importance of water to particular organ systems, however, is less understood by most people.

Research indicates that a thorough flushing of the mucus folds in the colonic tract (where toxins and wastes generally remain) will clean the system, and keep the body healthy and the immune system strong—which is essential in preventing and treating chronic pain and disease.

When you drink ample quantities of water, the colon becomes more effective, thus increasing the quantity and supply of fresh blood that can then move throughout your body, reducing toxic buildup while increasing pain relief.

By the same token, quantities of water are known to revitalize the kidneys and liver. I have already discussed the kidneys' functions relative to removing waste from the blood. To successfully remove that waste, the kidneys require water, which they use to properly filter toxins. Without enough water, the kidneys are not able to filter toxins from the bloodstream the way they should, leading to a host of health problems.

The kidneys are really the primary organs that regulate water balance within the body. As long as they have an ample supply of water, the kidneys manage this balance efficiently: excess water in the body is simply excreted as urine, easily returning to the body to proper balance.

When the body is dehydrated, however, the kidneys have a much harder job to do. They continue to try to filter the blood, but they have less water to use for the task. As a result, the kidneys generate more concentrated urine. This puts more stress and strain on the kidneys, which will harm kidney function over time.

Furthermore, as the dehydrated kidneys take on more strain, the liver takes over some of the kidney's functions, and normal liver functions—including metabolizing fat—suffer as a result.

How Hydration Affects Pain

Unfortunately, we rarely attribute the pain we feel to something as simple as a water shortage. But think about it. How much water are you really drinking during the day? And I mean water, not some other drink like soda, coffee, or juice that the body has to filter first. When was the last time you drank a full glass of water?

A deficiency of water affects the muscles and joints. Without adequate hydration, the natural lubrication within our joints begins to decrease. That's important, because as joints move, the bones are protected by the cushioning of cartilage, which itself requires adequate hydration. To use an analogy, just like an engine without adequate oil, joints that rub together without adequate lubrication will begin to deteriorate. Thankfully, this is fairly easy to avoid by simply drinking more water.

Our muscles, and really our entire bodies, are affected negatively by deficiencies in water. As our body's water supply declines, our skin and muscles begin to shrink, much like a dried-out grape. The dehydrated muscle fibers not only cause pain by straining the joints, but the shortened muscles affect movement, breed trigger points, and can send pain throughout the body.

Water is also one of the key factors in maintaining a healthy spine. As previously mentioned, between every vertebrae in our spine lies a disc, and these are our natural shock absorbers. This water-filled inner ring of discs holds about 75 percent of the spine's load, really bearing the weight of the body itself.

When there's not enough water in the body, this inner ring begins to contract, shifting the load to the weak outer ring. When this happens, the bulk of the load is supported by the spine and the vertebrae themselves. This can cause swelling, compressed nerves, and possibly disc rupture.

Headaches are another ailment that can often be fixed by drinking more water. Most people are conditioned to grab an over-the-counter pain medicine at the onset of a headache.

I'll go into far more detail on headaches and migraines in a later chapter, but one thing bears mentioning now. If you grab a full glass of water to down your pain pill, you may actually be doing as much to relieve your headache with the water itself as you are with the pill. Try drinking a tall glass of water and skipping the drug, and see how you feel.

How to Hydrate Properly

Water is the only substance that can properly hydrate the body. Note that I am talking about pure, clean, straight from the filtered source water here. Coffees and teas, carbonated sodas, or sugar-filled fruit drinks will not take care of your needs in the same way. Think of it this way: you don't take a bath in dirty water and expect to come out clean.

Only pure and simple water will keep you healthy and help the body eliminate many of the underlying triggers affecting your health daily.

So how much water is enough?

Much is written about the specific quantities of water needed for the body to function properly. Certainly, drinking a single glass of water at lunch or dinner will not do the job, even though that may actually be more pure water than many drink in today's society. While the FDA recommends six eight-ounce glasses of water per day, other experts suggest consuming eight ounces of water per twenty pounds of body weight.

While the exact recommendations vary, two things are clear. First, we're a chronically dehydrated culture, so everyone likely needs to drink more water. And second, having too much water will only lead you to the bathroom a few more times, so err on the side of too much rather than too little.

Many people believe that if we don't feel thirsty, we don't need more water. Nothing could be further from the truth. First, by the time we feel thirst, we're already quite dehydrated. Second, to some extent, our bodies adapt to the amount of water we consume, and therefore, they may be used to functioning at a chronically dehydrated level. So for someone who is chronically dehydrated, by the time they feel thirsty, they have needed more water for quite some time.

We also know that a few factors do require certain people to drink more than others. As mentioned above, someone who weighs more should be drinking more water. People with a higher activity level also require more water to replace fluids that are lost during exercise.

Many of us find ourselves sitting inactively at our desks for most of the day as a simple side effect of our jobs. It's easy to become dehydrated in this environment, so here's a tip I live by: if you sit at a computer several hours a day, make it a point to get up every hour and get another glass of water.

Sex, age, and location also play a role in how much water you need each day. For example, men typically require more water per day than women. As we get older, our bodies are less able to determine when we need more water, so older people should drink on a regular schedule, even if they're not particularly thirsty. People living in warm climates should likewise drink water more often.

Try drinking a full glass before you start your day in the morning and a full glass with dinner at night. Replace sugary soft drinks with water to reduce your calorie intake and to keep caffeine from emptying your body of the water it already has.

Get in the habit of taking water with you wherever you go. Try drinking it more often, and see how much it helps. It's a ridiculously simple solution and can quickly reduce certain types of chronic pain, as well as many other ailments, including headaches and muscle cramps.

One way to gauge your water intake is in the color of your urine. When the urine stream is clear, you are properly hydrated. The more yellow it is, the more water your body needs. When urine is dark orange, you are in great need of liquids and it may take a day or two to replenish the water to a point where the urine is again clear.

The caveat here is that certain supplements will change the color of your urine. So bear in mind, when taking supplements, that the first or second pass of urine afterward may be discolored. You should, therefore, space your supplements out (discussed later) to ensure a good gauge of hydration if you decide to use the "urine color" indicator, as opposed to drinking water based on weight.

Easy, Healthy, Free

When you are properly hydrated, your body actually feels light and clean. But more than that, you're flushing out a good part of the toxins that may very well be at the root of your pain or illness.

Consuming healthy amounts of water may not completely eliminate your condition, but when you do this in combination with the rest of the strategies covered in this book, it's very likely to help.

Water is easy, healthy, and free, so why not try it? It's nothing more than a habit. If you spend a week drinking more water, you will very likely find your body feeling better and craving the higher water intake. You have nothing to lose—and a lot of wellness to gain.

Another excellent way to gain wellness through diet is by supplementing with vitamins and minerals. But not all supplements are created equal. In the next chapter, I'll take you through the positive impact of healthy supplementation and show you how to tell the health-boosters apart from the frauds.

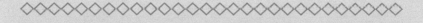

Chapter Review

- Water makes up roughly 75 percent of the human body (and 85 percent of the brain), and getting enough water every day is vital to your health and well-being.

- Water cleans out toxins, hydrates tissues and organs, regulates body temperature, and supplies oxygen, which is involved in nearly all chemical processes in the body.

- Lack of water affects the muscles and joints, causing them to rub together more closely, which can cause chronic pain and illness.

- Only pure and simple water will keep you healthy and help the body eliminate many of the underlying triggers affecting your health daily.

- While the FDA recommends six eight-ounce glasses of water per day, other experts suggest consuming eight ounces of water per twenty pounds of body weight.

Recommended Resources

Arthritis Reversed by Dr. Mark Wiley

You can get more information on the importance of hydration for joint pain and more in Dr. Mark Wiley's book, *Arthritis Reversed* at www.arthritisbookfree.com.

The 7-Day Back Pain Cure

I cover hydration as it relates specifically to back pain in more detail in my first book. You can get a free copy at www.losethebackpain.com

CHAPTER 14:

What Even the Healthiest Foods Are Still Missing

The Problem with Our Food Supply Today

One of the best pieces of advice I can give to anyone experiencing health problems is to eat a healthy, well-balanced diet. For many people, however, this seems to be a tall order. The good news is that it doesn't have to be, as you'll see here in this chapter.

These days, we see a lot of people making a greater effort to eat healthy. One common strategy there is to cut out fast food. But is this really helpful?

On the surface, yes. Fast food is loaded with unhealthy fats and excess sugars that should certainly be avoided. But what if I were to tell you that the actual nutritional value of your average fast food meal is not much different than that of a less-processed, home-cooked meal?

We often don't have time to cook homemade meals because we're on the go all the time. Even if we do take the time to slow things down and eat a home-cooked meal filled with a good amount of fruits and vegetables, unless they are organic or we grow them ourselves, we can never be sure of their nutritional content. And even then, most produce is grown in nutritionally depleted soil. This means that no matter how healthy you eat, you are still likely to have nutritional deficiencies.

This is scary, but true. Our food today lacks the mineral content that is needed for us to remain healthy. One reason for this is that the fruits and vegetables sold in stores aren't picked ripe. As a result, they lose up to 80 percent of the minerals that are absorbed during the ripening phase.

Mineral depletion in the food we eat is worsened by our current farming system, which often involves farming the same soil repeatedly without resting it every seven years, as our ancestors learned to do.

Instead of caring for the soil and replenishing its minerals, big business farms pour more and more fertilizers into their soil to get things to grow bigger and faster. And they build dams and levees to stop the natural flooding that has historically restored mineral content to the soil. These disastrous practices have been commonplace on US farms since the 1930s.

Think for a moment about what that means for the food we grow and consume today on US soil, which has become increasingly depleted of minerals over all that time. While we may be growing and eating something that looks like an ear of corn, its nutritional value is a far cry from what it used to be. Vegetables and fruits don't manufacture their own minerals. They get them from the soil. As soil loses minerals, so does the food grown from it.

The bottom line is simply this: current farming practices lead to mineral deficiencies in our soil, which leads to mineral deficiencies in the foods that we eat, and in turn, in our bodies.

That means we need to supplement our diets with the vitamins and minerals that are missing from our foods. This is a sad but true fact of life, and there is no way around it.

To best supplement your diet, at minimum, a high-quality multivitamin and a natural anti-inflammatory enzyme should be incorporated into your daily routine. In addition, we must ingest far more minerals in order to replace what has been lost from the soil and our modern foods.

Ideally, you should find out exactly what minerals your body is deficient in, and you should tailor a supplement plan that will bring you back to optimal health and homeostasis. We'll learn about this, and the rampant lies surrounding these key aspects of our health, in this chapter.

The Rise of Mineral Deficiencies

Unsurprisingly, given what we've just learned about the cause of mineral deficiency in our food supply, many of the diseases that we've come to think of as being a normal part of our lives did not even exist one hundred years ago. But the problem doesn't stop with the soil.

I have interviewed Dr. Robert Thompson, author of *The Calcium Lie* and *The Calcium Lie II* on several occasions, and he makes a very strong point regarding minerals. He reminds us that prior to the rise of refrigeration, the most common method of preserving meat, fish, and even vegetables, was to use sea salt.

Sea salt is 15 percent minerals. If we use sea salt all our lives, we're continually putting minerals back into our bodies. Since we're preserving food with refrigeration instead of sea salt, most of us consume far too little sea salt. Plus, due to the lies we've been told about salt intake, most of us do not consume enough salt, and rarely get the salt containing these needed minerals.

Sea salt not only contains the minerals we need, but is naturally iodized. Compare this to common table salt that has much of its natural mineral content removed, and is then iodized to replace just one of its missing minerals. Don't be taken in by the wrong-headed conventional "wisdom" that tells us we're all eating too much salt. The truth is, we're not eating enough of the *right* salt: sea salt.

Quality Multivitamins Are Critical

To give the body the nutrients it needs, everyone should take a high-quality multivitamin. I put a lot of emphasis on "high quality," because there are a lot of pills out there that aren't going to do you much good. Many companies manufacture products that are highly compressed and glued together into hard tablets that can be very difficult for the body to digest.

You can visualize this process. Imagine if you took a bunch of different vitamins in powder form and pressed them all together, slammed them flat, processed them through a bunch of machines, added binding ingredients to keep them together, sprinkled in preservatives so they would last for months on the shelf, and then spit this out as this hardened, rock-like pill.

That's how most multivitamins and supplements are produced. The less processing they go through, the better. The problem is, most people just look at the price and go for the cheapest brand. But in the world of supplements, you often get what you pay for.

Do you really want to pay for glue instead of vitamins and minerals in your supplement? If you want something that's actually going to help your body stay healthy, invest in a product that's highly digestible.

There are several ways to identify a highly digestible supplement. Most capsules—which are soft containers filled with the supplement itself—are easily digestible, especially those made from plant-based products that come from a reputable supplier. Soft-gel caplets are usually a good option as well, as they do not suffer from the squeeze and glue processing mentioned above.

Many manufacturers of high-quality supplements for single or small combinations of vitamins and minerals will also produce a pure liquid form of the supplement, which is also a very good option. And even though it's rare, there are a small handful of companies out there that actually do offer high-quality tablet-based supplements. However, because these exceptions to the rule are difficult to find, it's best to stick with capsules, caplets, or liquid forms of supplements when you can.

Because higher-quality, more easily digestible forms of supplements aren't made with high compression, you're probably going to have to take more pills to get a full dose. For example, if you don't smash and press all the nutrients together, they take up more volume, and so a full dose will have to be spread across multiple pills.

Keep in mind that in these cases, your vitamin dosage isn't necessarily higher, it's just uncompressed, which makes it much easier to digest. The vitamins are much more likely to be absorbed by your body. Remember, it's not how many vitamins you ingest that matters, it's how many your body can actually absorb and use.

Look for a quality multivitamin that *exceeds* the recommended daily allowance (RDA) of vitamins and minerals, as the RDA is severely inadequate for optimal heath. Also, be sure to understand the label, as the various regulations of the industry leave the door open for a lot of deception in the quest for greater profit at the expense of your health.

Vitamin Label Lies

Reading the supplement facts on vitamins can seem a little like a puzzle. This is in part because most "ingredients" are followed by some form of qualifier in parentheses. It's almost like they're listing two names for the same thing—only they're not.

When a vitamin label lists a vitamin or mineral followed by a parenthesis and the word "as," it's really telling you that it's not a real vitamin or mineral. This is the sneaky way that manufacturers are legally telling you that you're getting a synthetic attempt at recreating that vitamin or mineral. Another name for a synthetic, chemical compound designed to make us feel better is "a drug."

Be careful to avoid products with these ingredients when purchasing supplements. Not only will the body be unable to synthesize and use them as it would an actual vitamin or mineral, but you will also be exposing yourself to drug-like side effects.

The most common vitamin label lie that many fall victim to is that of vitamin C. We're all instructed, quite rightly, that vitamin C is a necessary supplement we should all be taking. However, since most products promoted as vitamin C are actually ascorbic acid, most of us aren't actually getting what we need.

Dr. Robert Thompson is very concerned about this and speaks out about it in his books and lectures across the country. He stresses how negligent it is that medical professionals continue to tout the importance of vitamin C, but then give patients the recommendation to take their "vitamin C (as ascorbic acid)."

He is adamant, and I agree, that you must take vitamin C that comes completely from whole food sources, such as organic fruits or vegetables. Taking any fake forms will not only leave you deficient, but may also cause other side effects like any other drug.

Be careful and informed when purchasing supplements. Make sure you read the label, and that you are really getting exactly what you need—not some lab's attempt to create a fake version of it.

Commonly Believed Nutrition Lies

Unfortunately, the current medical paradigm often lacks good awareness about supplements and their effects on our health. That means that even doctors who do try to address mineral deficiency by incorporating supplements into their practice are often guilty of misunderstanding and misusing them. Even worse, they pass along this bad information to their patients.

In turn, some of this bad information has become entrenched "medical wisdom" that the average person believes to be true—sometimes with dire consequences.

The Calcium Lie

Perhaps the biggest mistruth about supplements that most people in the US believe today is what medical practitioner and renowned author Dr. Robert Thompson refers to in his books as "the Calcium Lie."

In a nutshell, for years, consumers—especially women—have been led to believe calcium supplementation is an essential part of staying well as we age, and avoiding the mineral loss that leads to osteoporosis.

In truth, 90 percent of the US population actually has an *excess* of calcium relative to the amounts of other helpful minerals that are needed to make calcium useful to our bodies.

This excess calcium can have serious implications for our health, and has been associated with the shrinking of the brain, dementia, poisoned memory cells, higher rates of hyperthyroidism, weight gain, obesity and heart disease. In fact, we now know through meta-analysis that calcium supplementation increases the risk of heart disease by over 30 percent.

Clearly, supplementing with calcium alone can be dangerous. Yet this dangerous "medical wisdom" is still promoted, and many people believe it to be true. Countless Americans are still taking calcium supplements, or purchasing food fortified with calcium they don't need.

It's important to take the time to research and understand the other minerals that should be taken concurrently with calcium in order to avoid negative health risks. I'll talk more about this later in this chapter.

The Salt and Cholesterol Lie

Dr. Thompson warns us that another commonly believed mistruth is that we all ought to be watching our salt intake. In fact, this is among the most popular advice people get from their doctors. In truth, the vast majority of people need more salt, not less.

If you research the physiology of how sodium functions in the human body, you'll see that it plays an essential role in digesting protein and getting glucose and amino acid into every one of our cells—except for fat cells. In fact, hypertension is actually caused by *low* salt.

Still another example of a common nutritional belief that is wholly unfounded in science is this: How many people have been told by their doctors or other experts that if you're watching your cholesterol, you should avoid eating eggs? Just about everybody has heard this advice. In fact, egg yolk is the most similar to human protein of anything else we eat. That yolk is pure HDL (commonly termed "good") cholesterol, the same substance that makes up 25 percent of our brains.

There is no "bad" cholesterol or fat in eggs. That said, how you cook your eggs does make a difference, health-wise. What is the correct way to cook them? Never scramble your eggs. Scrambling causes the egg to become toxic, creating lipid peroxide fat. But as long as you're eating intact cooked egg yolk—over easy, or over hard—with that membrane still around it, then that egg is 100 percent healthy eating. If anything, most people should eat more eggs.

These are the most commonly believed nutritional lies that we've been fooled into believing. The so-called experts who taught us these things, even when they meant well, were simply mistaken.

Meanwhile, forward-thinking practitioners like Dr. Robert Thompson can tell you that—contrary to the conventional wisdom—their sickest patients often have an excess of calcium and a deficiency of salt.

This combination can be devastating for your health, causing problems like hypertension and worse.

The Truth about Calcium and Osteoporosis

I've established in this chapter that most of us have fallen prey to what Dr. Thompson terms "the calcium lie"—the idea that we're calcium deficient, when in truth, most of us have an excess of calcium in our bodies.

But what is the effect of this excess calcium? And if not through calcium supplementation, how do we avoid health concerns like osteoporosis?

First, let's turn to the numerous health problems associated with excess calcium. These include kidney stones, gall stones, bone spurs, plaque, calcium deposits, cataracts, brain shrinkage and dysfunction, as well as heart disease, hardening of the arteries, dementia, cancer, diabetes, hypothyroidism, and over 90 percent of hypertension. In particular, it is believed by experts who study these issues that the combination of low sodium and high calcium may be a leading cause of hypertension.

Several large-scale studies have shown a direct connection between calcium supplementation and its impact on heart health. In 2010, meta-analysis of multiple large studies encompassing over eight thousand people showed a 31 percent increase in the incidence of heart attacks for those who took 500 mg of calcium per day. Since this amount of calcium is actually lower than the average bottle sold in stores, the dangers of calcium supplementation should be very clear.

Unfortunately, the dangers extend beyond heart attacks. Eleven other studies all found a 20 percent increase in strokes linked with calcium supplementation, and strokes and sudden death taken together increased 18 percent.

Yet in spite of this information, well-meaning but uninformed doctors and media outlets are still telling people to increase their calcium intake.

Dr. Thompson has established that "make sure you get your calcium" does not work as a means of avoiding osteoporosis. Not only that, but clearly taking too much calcium comes with the added risk of a variety of serious health problems. Calcium doesn't help your bones, nor does it "do a body good." On the contrary, as you've just seen, excess calcium and calcium supplementation actually lead to heart attack, stroke, and other deadly and debilitating illnesses for most people.

We cannot replace the minerals our bodies need by calcium alone, because it is only one of several needed for bone health. Instead, we must find other methods of doing this, such as consuming sea salt, as covered in the previous pages.

It is unfortunate, but the medical industry's current approach to detecting and treating osteoporosis is all wrong. Their mistake lies in accepting the idea that it is normal or expected for there to be a decline in the mineral levels in our bodies as we advance in age.

The established medical "wisdom" has, to date, chiefly concerned itself with merely measuring and documenting the mineral deficiency across the entire aging population when in fact, osteoporosis is a completely preventable nutritional disease—and a modern one at that. I'll talk more about osteoporosis in chapter 19.

Protecting Your Bones and Joints

A common worry for many of us, both young and old, is the continued strength of our bones and joints. Eating the best, wholesome foods and staying hydrated will go a long way toward maintaining healthy bones. But first, here are the specific supplements you should look into in order to support your bone and joint health, first covered by Dr. Mark Wiley in his book, *Arthritis Reversed*, and reproduced with permission below.

Rebuilding Bone and Cartilage

Avocado Soybean Unsaponifiables (ASU)
ASU is a vegetable extract made from the oil of avocados and soybeans that is said to slow the progression of osteoarthritis. It does this by slowing down the production of inflammatory chemicals in the body and thus the breakdown of cartilage in the joints. It has also been found to spur new cartilage cell growth. ASU is available in capsule form at a recommended 300 mg daily.

Chondroitin Sulfate
Within the cartilage around your joints is a chemical known as chondroitin. Chondroitin is naturally produced by the body, but as you age, your natural supply starts to plummet. A loss of chondroitin from the cartilage is linked to a major cause of joint pain. What's more, through wear and tear, this can lead joint cartilage to break down, resulting in the condition of osteoarthritis.

We can't regenerate cartilage on our own, but we can take a supplement called chondroitin sulfate that has been shown by studies to help slow down this degenerative process and reduce arthritic pain. Chondroitin sulfate is made from the cartilage of cows and other animals, and is often used in combination with other products, including glucosamine and manganese.

Hydrolyzed Collagen Type 2

Collagen—particularly type 2 collagen—is the main structural building block of joint cartilage. The human body is made up of 60 percent type 2 collagen, and hydrolyzed type 2 collagen contains the amino acids found in human cartilage. Your body uses these amino acids to create new collagen, and to repair the cartilage and connective tissue throughout your body. Hydrolyzed collagen type 2 also contains hyaluronic acid, which lubricates your joints.

Vitamin D3

Vitamin D3 is a fat-soluble vitamin that promotes calcium absorption and enables normal mineralization and growth of the bones. Deficiency of vitamin D3 (the active source of vitamin D) can lead to loss of bone density and brittle or misshapen bones. Ample levels can help prevent osteoporosis. It is important that you ask your healthcare provider to test your vitamin D blood levels, to ensure you do not get too much.

Lubricating Joints

Cetyl Myristoleate (CMO)

Cetyl myristoleate (CMO) is an ethylated esterified fatty acid derived from bovine tallow oil. Though it is similar to fish oil, it is made specifically to help joints through its action as a cellular lubricant. Clinical studies show CMO to be an effective anti-inflammatory compound that promotes healthy joint function. It increases joint flexibility and range of motion by lubricating the joint at a cellular level.

CMO works to decrease inflammation in the joints and to lubricate their movement. In other words, it increases the fluids that cushion the space between the bones in your joints. CMO is reported to effect change at the cellular level, within the cell membranes themselves. It assists in the reduction and prevention of breakdown in joint cartilage.

Methylsulfonylmethane (MSM)

MSM is a potent sulfur naturally found in plants, animals, and humans, and it helps rebuild the connective tissue in your joints. What's more, MSM has the unique ability to improve cell permeability. This allows harmful toxins to flow out, and health-boosting nutrients to flow in to feed your joints, cartilage, and connective tissue.

MSM is used for hundreds of symptoms related to a myriad of health diseases and conditions, and is especially effective at relieving inflammation for improved joint function, and pain associated with joint inflammation, osteoarthritis, rheumatoid arthritis, osteoporosis, and tendonitis. One study published in the *Journal of Anti-Aging Medicine* found that MSM provides an 80 percent greater reduction in pain compared to a placebo.

Fish Oil and Omega 3 Fatty Acids
The omega-3 fatty acids found in abundance in fish oil derived from cod, trout, herring, salmon, and other cold-water fish are proven to reduce inflammation. Research from Cardiff University in Great Britain found that cod liver oil not only relieves pain, but also stops and even reverses the damage caused by osteoarthritis and rheumatoid arthritis. Omega-3s help morning stiffness, regenerate joint tissue, and have been shown to also aid in autoimmune disease like RA, lupus, and psoriasis.

According to recommendations of the Arthritis Foundation, when treating conditions related to arthritis it is best to use "fish oil capsules with at least 30 percent EPA/ DHA, the active ingredients. For lupus and psoriasis, 2 grams EPA/DHA three times a day. For Raynaud's phenomenon, 1 gram four times a day. For rheumatoid arthritis, up to 2.6 grams fish oil (1.6 grams EPA) twice a day."

Natural Anti-Inflammatory Enzymes

Our modern-day diet, full of processed and nutritionally void foods, triggers an increase of inflammation in our bodies, until we're overloaded with it—an excess. Inflammation creates pain in our muscles, nerves, and joints, and is always a big factor in all kinds of chronic pain and illness.

What we need is more of the nutrients that cool inflammation down (found in fruits, vegetables, nuts, and fish) and more of our own natural anti-inflammatories—the proteolytic enzymes that stop inflammation and clear out scar tissue. Unfortunately, most of us aren't eating enough anti-inflammatory nutrients, and as we get older, our bodies make fewer anti-inflammatory enzymes.

Enzymes are basically the main line of defense against inflammation. Enzymes are not anti-inflammatory drugs, but they reduce inflammation by neutralizing the bio-chemicals of inflammation to levels where the creation, repair, and regeneration of injured tissues can take place.

Reducing inflammation can have an immediate impact on improved heart health, cancer prevention and recovery, and Alzheimer's prevention. It also helps speed up recovery from sprains, strains, fractures, bruises, contusions, surgery, and arthritis. Systemic enzymes work to reduce inflammation and promote healing without any side effects. Plus, Dr. Nicholas Gonzalez has found great success in treating cancer using these enzymes, which we'll cover in a later chapter.

So, first, as mentioned, you need to eat a healthy diet and take a quality multivitamin in order to give your body the nutrients needed to counteract the inflammation response. Second, you need to replenish the body with more of its own natural anti-inflammatory enzymes. When you do this, two things happen: You cool inflammation and you clear out the stiffened scar tissue that it leaves behind. That means less pain and more fluidity in movement, since scar tissue is what makes us feel stiff in the first place.

It's best to find a supplement that combines enzymes and herbs in a formula targeted to reduce inflammation and pain. Look at the "other ingredients" listed below the supplement facts and avoid animal derivatives, preservatives, or artificial things like titanium dioxide. Finally, as with multivitamins, look for capsules or gel tabs.

If you suffer from any sort of aches or pain, or if you just want to get and stay as healthy as possible, you should consider systemic enzymes. They have been used to safely and effectively eliminate pain and inflammation from all sorts of conditions like arthritis, colitis, back pain, sciatica, joint pain, heart disease, cancer, and more.

The enzyme formula I recommend is Heal-n-Soothe, which contains the highest concentration of enzymes and several other pain-relieving herbs, and can be found at www.losethebackpain.com/healnsoothe.

The ingredients in this formula have tons of clinical studies behind them, as well as hundreds of years of use, so it's a safer bet than a lot of others on the market. It also has numerous other herbs, vitamins, and nutrients that have been proven to have anti-inflammatory effects and, together, they make an extremely effective combination.

Supplement Your Life

In your quest for a healthy life, adding supplements to a wholesome diet is just plain smart. Again, make sure you know how to read supplement labels so you can verify that what you're taking is natural and effective. By finding the right multivitamin and helping your body replenish its natural anti-inflammatory enzymes, you can rebuild your natural state of homeostasis and ensure that your body is getting all of its needs met.

While a quality multivitamin makes a great start to a healthy supplementation regimen, it's an even stronger choice to create a supplement program that is specifically tailored to your own body's needs.

How to Correctly Use Supplements

Before you start taking mineral supplements, it's important to understand a few key strategies and truths. First on this list is understanding whether or not you actually need some or all of the minerals available as supplements. Second, you must identify what types of minerals you do need, how each mineral was derived, and which ones are the best for you.

Let's start with identifying quality mineral supplements. There are three types of minerals available to supplement our diets. They are ionic, chelate, and colloidal minerals, and are summarized nicely by Dr. Thompson in his book, *The Calcium Lie II*.

Ionic minerals are those in salt form that your body can actually use. In fact, sea salt has every mineral that humans need for optimal health. The fact that they come in ionic form means that they are natural, unprocessed, and readily available for effective absorption. Chemically, they conduct electricity, can dissolve completely in water, and most importantly, they can cross cell membranes and donate electrons.

This is important because electrons are needed to fuel all of the chemical reactions that take place in the body to keep it working. Adding ionic minerals to your supplement regime—even with something as simple as pure sea salt—will unquestionably take your health to the next level.

Unlike ionic minerals, chelated minerals are not pure. This is because they basically come in rock form, which means they have amino acids attached. Because of their structure, if your body actually needs a particular chelated mineral, these can be beneficial. However, unless you are certain you need a particular mineral, taking them unnecessarily can contribute to imbalance in the body, causing harm rather than a benefit to your health.

In the past, there was a lot of talk about colloidal minerals, with little public understanding of what they actually were. Colloidal minerals are essentially worthless, and in fact, they can even be dangerous. This is because they do not conduct electricity and can't cross cell membranes, and both of these missing qualities are needed if a mineral is to have any impact on the body's health.

What's more, since they can't enter cells, colloidal minerals stay between cells, where they accumulate over time, leading to a whole host of other problems.

Osteoporosis is typically thought of as being caused by loss of calcium from our bones, but this is an oversimplification that totally misses the mark. In truth, it's the loss of many needed minerals from our bones—not just calcium. Common treatments for osteoporosis include weight-burning exercise, calcium, vitamin D, hormone, estrogen, calcitonin, bisphosphonate drugs, and other drugs. But what patients really need to do is to make sure they're getting their minerals.

I commonly hear from people who think they don't need to supplement with additional minerals because there are minerals present in their daily vitamins. What they often don't realize is that these minerals are generally chelated. Plus, in a one-size-fits-all daily vitamin, you are likely getting minerals you are not actually deficient in along with the ones you need, which causes imbalance in your body.

This truth that one size does not fit all is perhaps the most important thing to understand here. Your approach to mineral supplements should never be "all or none." In the same way that eating excess food when you're not hungry can lead to pain and weight gain, excesses of unnecessary minerals will lead to imbalances and health problems. Find out what your body is actually deficient in before taking supplements you don't need, which can harm your health.

Know Your Mineral Levels, Know Better Health

The best way to get an analysis of what the mineral levels in your body are is to use micro mass spectrometry. A better-known name for this type of testing is hair tissue mineral analysis (HTMA). Unfortunately, many medical professionals look down their noses at this method because they are ignorant of its benefits.

This technology is reliable. It is used by every chemistry lab in the world and has even been used to determine the mineral content of the soil on Mars. It can help you figure out if your body is in mineral imbalance, and it can show you the path back to homeostasis. Seek out this testing on your own. There are many reputable, expert labs that offer it around the country.

Once you know what you're deficient in, and conversely, have an excess of, you'll know which supplements to take and which to avoid. This is the key to using supplements smartly and safely.

Now you know how increasing your intake of vitamins and minerals can take your health to a completely new level of homeostasis. But how do you get rid of the toxins in your system that have built up over time, so that those minerals can have their greatest impact? The next chapter will walk you through the importance of cleanses as the final piece in this diet pillar of the Complete Healing Formula™.

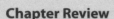

Chapter Review

- We need to supplement our diets with the vitamins and minerals that are missing from our foods.

- To best supplement your diet, at minimum, a high-quality multivitamin and a natural anti-inflammatory enzyme should be incorporated into your daily routine.

- Your multivitamin should be of high quality, or it will not give you the benefits you need.

- When a vitamin label lists a vitamin or mineral followed by a parenthesis and the word "as," it's really telling you that it's not a real vitamin or mineral.

- You can and should replenish the body with more of its own natural anti-inflammatory enzymes.

- About 90 percent of the US population actually has too much calcium relative to the amounts of other helpful minerals that are needed to make calcium useful to our bodies.

- Numerous health problems are associated with excess calcium, including kidney stones, gall stones, bone spurs, plaque, calcium deposits, cataracts, brain shrinkage and dysfunction, heart disease, hardening of the arteries, dementia, cancer, diabetes, and hypothyroidism.

- The foods we eat today are depleted of minerals as a result of the current farming system, which often involves farming the same soil repeatedly without resting it every seven years.

- To get the greatest health benefits, find out what your body is actually deficient in before taking supplements.

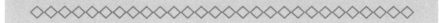

Recommended Resources

Hair Tissue Mineral Analysis

Dr. Robert Thompson, author of *The Calcium Lie*, recommends this non-invasive lab test to determine your mineral levels before taking any vitamin or mineral supplement.

Learn more at www.losethebackpain.com/mineral-analysis.

The Calcium Lie II by Dr. Robert Thompson

Get a free copy of Dr. Thompson's book, *The Calcium Lie II*, to learn more about your vitamin and mineral needs and what you can do about them. This book is my gift to you. Just visit www.losethebackpain.com/calcium-lie.

CHAPTER 15:

When Was the Last Time You Changed Your Oil?

An "Oil Change" for Your Health

Your body's process of maintaining the purity of your internal liquids is one its main functions. Picture the fluids in your body as a sewer system that collects the waste that your trillions of cells generate. Not only are millions of dead cells discarded into the blood and lymph system daily, so are several toxins that enter the body via the respiratory paths, digestive system, and skin.

In previous chapters, I discussed the importance of hydration as one of the ways the body keeps itself clean. But there's more to achieving and maintaining a clean system than just drinking water—especially after months and years of toxin buildup.

Cleansing is a critical part of the Wellness Model of Health™ because of the role it plays in balancing our systems. Several of our organs are designed specifically to cleanse our bodies. The intestines, liver, kidneys, skin, lungs, and lymphatic system are known as the emunctories, or detoxification organs.

During normal function, the amount of waste isn't more than the body can process, and the body stays clean. However, if the volume of waste is more than the emunctories can process, the organs aren't able to function as well and, slowly, the body becomes filled with toxins.

Undergoing a significant cleanse can have a tremendous impact on your chronic pain or illness, and can move you closer to achieving homeostasis by leaps and bounds. The number of cleanses needed will vary depending on your age, as well as several other conditions.

Dr. Hulda Clark has developed a number of protocols for kidney, liver, and intestine cleanses. Her books outline in detail cleanses that will help your organs return to their normal, homeostatic functions of cleansing and detoxifying your system of excesses, deficiencies, and stagnations.

I highly recommend that you locate a copy of one of Clark's books for the specific cleanse recipes, as this information is invaluable, yet far too lengthy for me to reproduce here. In this chapter, I'll focus on discussing the fundamentals of kidney, liver, and colon cleanses and how they work to restore your body to its most efficient state.

Cleanse Your Kidneys

We're all familiar with the body's most common form of toxic removal—urination. Our white blood cells are normally purged of toxins in the kidneys, sending those toxins downstream to the bladder. Much of this toxicity is then expelled in the urine. However, since the detoxification process starts at the kidneys, the kidneys themselves must be able to function properly—something that can't happen if they are already loaded with toxins in the first place.

Our white blood cells can't discard their load of toxins if our kidneys are loaded with toxins to begin with, which will keep our immune systems out of balance and suppressed. Dr. Clark recommends a kidney cleanse a minimum of once per year for three weeks for immune system recovery. Just like a dirty furnace filter will stop cleaning the air by just continuing to circulate the same pollutants we're looking to remove, the same is true with the kidneys. Clean kidneys can clean our systems; dirty kidneys make our systems dirty.

As you know, white blood cells are a critical part of our immune systems. For many individuals, and especially for those suffering from degenerative or chronic illnesses, the white blood cells are diseased with immunosuppressive agents including radioactivity, heavy metals, benzene, asbestos, PCBs, and azo dyes. The kidneys must be able to remove these agents from the blood in order for the afflicted individual to have hope of recovery.

In chapter 11, I detailed how these agents surround us in our daily lives. They are in our food, our water—even our cosmetics. That means that even those of us who have the normal amount of white blood cells should cleanse, because though the number of cells might be right, the quality of them might not. If our white blood cells are poisoned, they can't function and they can't combat viruses, bacteria, and other pathogens found in disease.

The kidneys also play an important role in regulating arterial pressure. They are a part of the hormonal process that regulates blood pressure and long-term extracellular volume. So you can look at a kidney cleanse as a step to regulate your blood pressure.

In its early stages, it is easy not to notice if your kidneys aren't functioning properly. A number of disorders result from your kidneys losing their function, such as skin, rheumatic, and circulatory disorders. Yet, as Dr. Clark points out, it is not common for doctors to consider kidney function when prescribing treatment. Again, most doctors are addressing the symptoms, not seeking the root cause of the illnesses, which very often lies in the kidneys.

One example is cardiovascular health, which isn't possible if the kidneys aren't functioning at a maximum. In their exposure to toxic substances, the kidneys are very susceptible to illness. Our entire body's health relies on a toxin-free system, which depends greatly on the kidneys.

A massive mobilization of toxins is often the result of cleansing and regularly prescribed parasite treatments. This can overload the kidney with many undesirable results. Dr. Clark says it is crucial to follow a kidney cleanse protocol to get the kidneys strong enough to accommodate the detoxifying and excretory capacity. Full details on the best way to begin and follow a kidney cleanse can be found in her book, or you can research the specifics online.

Cleanse Your Liver

While kidney function is very important, no organ has more functions in the body than the liver. So it's no surprise that your liver is your largest organ, weighing up to four pounds. The portal vein connects the liver to the digestive tract. During digestion, both nutrients and the toxins make their way to the liver via the portal vein. The liver functions to protect the rest of our organs by acting as a barrier and retaining dangerous elements.

The following are a few functions of the liver:

- It acts as a tank for our nutrients like iron, copper, and vitamins A and B12.

- It offers endless glucose to dependent tissues like the nervous system, erythrocytes, bone marrow, retina, and lymphocytes. It also has a nonstop capacity to synthesize glucose. While glycogen deposits in our muscles can greatly exceed those deposits in the liver, they are used solely as fuel for muscular contractions.

- It transforms the hemoglobin from our dead or dying red blood cells into bilirubin, and stores any excess iron to be used later.

- It produces bile, which is vital for proper digestion and absorption of fats. Bile contains acids that protect the intestinal mucosa so that if the bile doesn't flow as it should, the intestinal mucosa deteriorates, allowing bacteria to pass on to other organs. Bile functions as a laxative, excreting toxins, medicines, hormones, cholesterol, and more. It neutralizes toxins, and regulates cholesterol and steroid hormones. It also synthesizes nonessential amino acids and coagulation factors. This indicates that excessive bleeding could indicate liver impairment.

Dr. Clark recommends the following steps for improving liver function:

1. Do a bowel cleanse to eliminate parasites and correct dysbiosis and excess intestinal permeability.

2. The Ascaris Parasite Program. (See *The Cure for All Diseases* by Dr. Hulda Clark.)

3. Do a complete kidney cleanse.

4. Continue to do liver cleanses until no stones are yielded following three cleanses.

Our liver is like a lab, processing thousands of substances every second. It neutralizes a number of toxins so that the body can easily excrete them through urine or stool following digestion. Our enzyme system enables it to process endless toxins with a variety of substrates. When the liver can't detoxify properly, the rest of our organs suffer. Dr. Clark says that the only diseases that can't be relieved by liver function stimulation are congenital disorders.

Why Does the Liver Need Cleansing?

I've covered what the liver does, and we know that its purpose is to absorb harmful elements in the body. If that's the case, why does it need to be cleansed?

The biggest motive for cleansing the liver is to replenish its ability to clean and detoxify our bodies. This protocol also rids the gallbladder of gallstones, which contain pathogens that make them continuously susceptible to reinfection. While our blood tests might show normal levels of transaminases, this only is an indication of liver destruction rather than liver cleanliness or functionality. Throughout our lives, we commonly overwhelm our livers with residue and pathogens.

Bile doesn't just emulsify fat in the intestine, it also prevents bacteria growth in the digestive tract and stimulates peristalsis—the body's natural process to move digestive waste through our systems. This is why people who suffer from liver issues or a lazy gallbladder are overly gassy or constipated.

If not drained adequately every day, the bile ducts and gallbladder will hold onto cholesterol and form stones. This in turn results in a hindrance of further drainage, creating a vicious cycle. This leads to the production of cholestasis and the stagnation of bile flow, creating hepatic congestion that disturbs proper venous circulation, digestion, and excretion of toxins.

A congested liver is the cause of many instances of dermatitis, fatigue, joint pain, headaches, depression, indigestion, sinusitis, bleeding gums, forehead wrinkles, and more.

Stones don't just form in the gallbladder, they also form in the liver ducts. The liver is comprised of several ducts, so when a stone gets trapped in one of them, the hepatic lobes can't drain and the whole body feels the impacts. Dr. Clark advises ingesting olive oil and grapefruit juice to help discharge bile by releasing these stones.

Epsom salts are used in Dr. Clark's liver cleanse to help relax the liver and intestine while dehydrating parasites.

Many of the stones that accumulate in our liver go undetected by traditional medicine because their density is similar to our tissues. They must be calcified to be seen, and thus aren't detectable in MRIs, ultrasounds, or X-rays. However, the stones in the gallbladder are calcified and can be seen with those tests.

Dr. Clark recommends the following tips prior to doing a liver cleanse:

- If you have impaired kidney function, you should not do a liver cleanse. If you are unsure, there are home kits you can use to test your urinary albumin, which are useful for early kidney dysfunction detection.

- You also should not do a cleanse if it doesn't help excrete gallstones and gallbladder sludge.

- You need to fast for fourteen hours prior to the cleanse so that there are no intestinal obstructions.

- For ultimate effectiveness, avoid consuming fats on the day of the cleanse.

- Put your feet up between five o'clock and nine o'clock in the evening, or massage them to help detoxify the lymphatic system.

- If possible, ozonate the oil for twenty minutes.

- Only do the cleanse if you are in good health, as you will need energy.

Following the cleanse, Dr. Clark advises to continue regular waste excretion by emptying your bowels.

Cleanse Your Colon

Although the term "colon cleanse" suggests a focus on just the colon, most effective colon cleanses really target your digestive system as a whole. They address the excesses, deficiencies, and stagnations in that whole area of your body's system.

When food is not fully digested, it becomes stagnant in your digestive tract—most often in the colon. This creates an atmosphere that invites the accumulation of toxins, parasites, and inflammation. But while the undigested food is a problem that must be cleared, the bigger problem actually starts earlier in the chain of digestion.

Many of our digestive problems start in our stomachs. Many people today are deficient in hydrochloric acid (HCl), which is an essential part of digestion. Not only does this acid begin to break down our food, it also is critical in eliminating many of the parasites and pathogens that may enter our bodies along with our food. Unfortunately, much of the medical and pharmaceutical community seems to be on a mission to remove HCl from our bodies.

Dr. Thompson showed in his book, *The Calcium Lie II*, that the steady climb in indigestion and heartburn that we've been experiencing as a culture are a direct result of the recommendations to limit our salt intake. Our bodies are unable to generate the appropriate levels of stomach acid when minerals like salt are deficient. As a result, we do not have enough HCl to digest properly.

Worse, the deficiency of HCl in the stomach allows bacteria and other invaders to flourish in our stomachs. Dr. Clark explained that this results in acidity or reflux in the esophagus. Rather than battling the cause of the reflux by allowing the stomach acid to increase, modern medicine douses all HCl through the use of antacids, thereby creating a self-fulfilling prophecy. Deficiencies of stomach acid then feed the excess of bacteria, which ultimately leads to stagnation—a clogged colon.

That clogged colon then leads to inflammation of the gastrointestinal tract, causing a condition that's known as "leaky gut." This condition allows toxins from the waste in your bowel to leak into your blood stream. Not only can the colon become clogged with anywhere between five to twenty pounds of hardened fecal matter, it can also reduce your gastrointestinal tract's ability to synthesize and absorb key nutrients into your blood stream to promote healthy brain and organ function.

You can stop this problem from happening by managing your diet, keeping toxins to a minimum, and ingesting enough sea salt. But most people also need to conduct regular colon cleanses to ensure a properly functioning system.

Cleaning House

Think of cleanses the way you think about your normal housekeeping schedule. Cleanses are necessary to keep things running smoothly, and the more often you clean, the easier it is to achieve homeostasis. Following Dr.

Clark's advice for cleansing your vital organs will ensure that they continue to work hard and smart for you, giving you a long, healthy, and clean life.

I've shown you all the building blocks you need to construct your health from a mental, physical, and diet standpoint. But what if you or someone you love is already suffering from an ailment caused by the lack of homeostasis in any of these three key areas? The next several chapters will provide specific recommendations for some of the most prevalent ailments in the US today, including migraines, arthritis, chronic back pain, osteoporosis, fibromyalgia, heart disease, and cancer.

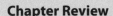

Chapter Review

- Cleansing is a critical part of our health, helping to remove millions of dead cells discarded into the blood and lymph system daily along with toxins.

- The intestines, liver, kidneys, skin, lungs, and lymphatic system are known as the emunctories, or detoxification organs.

- Undergoing a significant cleanse can have a tremendous impact on your chronic pain or illness.

- Kidney and liver cleanses are excellent ways to improve your health and wellness.

- Colon cleanses are essential to proper digestion, improved nutrition, and avoiding chronic illnesses.

- The more often you cleanse, the easier it will be to keep your systems running smoothly.

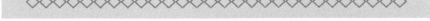

Recommended Resources

Dr. Clark Research Association

Learn more about the tools available to clear these toxins from your system from the Dr. Clark Research Association at www.drclark.com.

Clark Therapy by Ignacio Chamorro Balda

You can also get more information and details on the tools and methods based on Dr. Clark's work in the book *Clark Therapy* by Ignacio Chamorro Balda.

Natural Cleanse

A product I strongly recommend to keep your colon health regular is called Natural Cleanse. You can get it from Living Well Nutraceuticals at http://livingwellnutraceuticals.com.

PART II:

The End of All Disease

CHAPTER 16:

The End of Migraines

What Are Migraines?

Have you ever made up a headache as an excuse to get out of something? Next time, try using a migraine instead. Migraines will get you out of anything—whether you want to go or not. Not only are migraines debilitating to many who suffer from them, but these—and their evil twin, the chronic headache—can result in considerable suffering and a loss of productivity.

Dr. Mark Wiley studied migraines extensively in his book, *Outwitting Headaches,* which he wrote after struggling with migraines himself for years. Think of the migraine as an angrier, more severe, and more persistent version of an average headache. More than that, Dr. Wiley notes that migraines often come with a host of other symptoms, such as dizziness and vomiting. Those who suffer from migraines know that they can take a terrible toll on your daily life, undermining your natural homeostasis and the entire Wellness Model of Health™.

Migraine headaches are caused by both vasoconstriction and dilation, which means the blood vessels are either constricting or they are expanding. This is that throbbing sensation you feel sometimes if you have a headache, more like a drum beat versus a tight, squeezing feeling.

This chapter will cover the myths, lies, and truths about migraines, as well as effective treatment and prevention methods.

The Myths and Lies of Migraines

Migraines are powerful and painful occurrences that can severely disrupt your daily life. When it comes to this serious condition, it's best to be able to discern what's true and what isn't about your suffering.

Myth: Medicine Will Fix the Problem

One common misperception about migraines is that you can treat it with a pill. But as Dr. Wiley points out, you will never win the migraine war by dealing with the pain once you already feel it or by taking a pill to prevent it. You are only putting off the pain and creating a diversion.

The only way to be victorious against migraines is prevention. You need to learn what the causes are and change your lifestyle accordingly.

When a migraine occurs, there are a lot of negative things happening to your body that you aren't aware of. Taking medication, both over-the-counter and prescribed, just masks the pain and prevents you from feeling the migraine. Whatever triggered it is still there, however, and could, unbeknown to you, even be affecting your health. Remember, pain is the body's way of alerting us to a problem, and masking it only hides the real cause of the issue—it doesn't make it go away.

There are negative consequences to medication as well, and the best way to become migraine-free is to get to the root of your pain and make changes to your life to prevent them from returning.

Myth: Coffee Is a Cure

Another myth is that a cup of coffee is a great fix for a migraine. Coffee is a diuretic, which causes you to urinate and sweat. Caffeine also has toxins in it, not to mention the sugar, cream, and artificial sweeteners often added to your morning cup. As Dr. Wiley explains, all of these things lead to dehydration and elevated sugar levels, which makes coffee a poor choice for someone looking to avoid migraines.

In fact, many people who suffer headaches don't know that their caffeine consumption is actually causing their migraines in the first place. I learned this in my own personal experience back in the day, when I drank too much coffee each day at the office.

Once I stopped drinking coffee and tea, I started to realize that I always got a headache after I got home from work. At first I thought it was the kids, but no: I discovered that I was actually suffering from caffeine withdrawal. After this realization, I switched to decaffeinated tea, and my consistent headaches were gone in days.

True Causes of Migraines

There are many reasons why we get migraines. Genetics and environmental factors are some of the causes. The other causes are more like triggers. The good news is that triggers can be avoided by making simple adjustments to your lifestyle so a migraine-free existence is not out of your reach.

Dehydration

As I mentioned previously, your body is 75 percent water and your brain is over 85 percent water. Water is the fluid of blood, ridding the body of toxins through breathing, sweating, and urinating. In your kidneys, impure fluids present in the body get separated out from the pure fluids, and the filtered toxins get sent to your bladder.

I've covered the importance of water as it relates to removing toxins from our systems, but it also has a direct impact on the constriction, or lack thereof, in our blood vessels. When you become dehydrated, the body can't supply the vital organs with the quality cleansing and fortifying blood it needs—a deficiency that is marked by telltale headaches. That means that inadequate hydration can and will prime your system for a migraine.

As I mentioned earlier, you can easily tell if you're dehydrated by paying attention to your urine. It should be pale yellow, and if it's a darker yellow or orange, you are very dehydrated. Migraine sufferers should be especially vigilant in checking their urine, as hydration is necessary for prevention.

Oxygen Deprivation

Blood carries oxygen through your body. People tend to breathe from the top of their lungs, only getting 60 percent of the oxygen they need. This also means they are likely exhaling less, which could lead to a 60 percent increase in carbon dioxide in the body.

According to Dr. Wiley, a lack of proper oxygen to the brain creates poor bodily function—something we've all experienced in the feeling of lightheadedness.

But it also can lead to migraines for those who are more prone to suffer from them.

Sleep Deprivation

As I discussed in chapter 4, sleep is a time for your body to repair itself, and we produce serotonin while we sleep. Dr. Wiley found that one of the causes of migraines is a deficiency of serotonin, so it's logical that not getting enough sleep contributes to migraines.

Not only is your body repairing itself during sleep, but it is also detoxing. While you breathe and sweat overnight, your body's cells reproduce and your liver cleans your blood. Then, when you take your morning shower, you clean off the detoxed materials you've sweated out. Without a good night's sleep, you are robbing your body of its ability to detox. The more toxins you have, the more migraines you get.

So what's the first thing you probably do when you're tired? You reach for caffeine. Coffee, soda, black tea, even pills. As I mentioned earlier, Dr. Wiley clearly states that coffee and caffeine can lead to dehydration, which has already been discussed as a trigger. The cure for a deficiency of sleep is sleep, pure and simple.

Exercise

According to Dr. Wiley, a proper exercise routine is very important for migraine sufferers. If you have a headache, the last thing you want to do is hit the treadmill. However, if you don't exercise, you aren't reducing your stress, increasing your blood flow, or increasing your oxygen intake. All three of these factors have been identified as migraine triggers.

Migraine sufferers should establish an exercise routine. Start by walking and gently swinging your arms to get your limbs moving and the oxygen and heart pumping. Gentle yoga, tai chi, and QiGong are all good options for you to exercise and stretch.

Diet

Dr. Wiley's research also found that diet is a main offender when it comes to migraines. Foods like hamburgers, cheese, pizza, lunchmeats, and milk are all staples for many American households. Unfortunately, these foods have a high concentration of nitrates, which can trigger a migraine immediately.

Let's say you eat chicken *parmagiana* for dinner. To start with, the chicken is breaded and fried. Even if you use olive oil, too much concentration of any oil can obstruct the channels where the blood moves, affecting your breathing, and in turn, leading to possible oxygen deprivation, another trigger. The sugar in the breading can raise your blood sugar and blood fat levels, which can ultimately lead to migraines. Plus, the cheese in this dish, like any dairy animal milk product, can cause headaches and affect your fat levels, which also leads to headaches.

Other foods to avoid include anything fermented, such as pickles or other pickled foods. While fermented foods are excellent for your health under normal circumstances, if you suffer from migraines, removing them from your diet may offer you relief.

As I identified at the start of this book, imbalances in the body that stem from excesses, deficiencies, or stagnation can cause headaches, and these imbalances can become apparent in the mind, body, and diet. With so many migraine triggers permeating the common American diet, combined with the stressors of our modern life, it's no wonder that so many people suffer from migraines.

Effective Treatment and Prevention for Migraines

Try this technique of Dr. Wiley's to give yourself some pain relief from migraines:

For a pounding migraine, fill up your sink all the way with hot water. Stick your hands into the water, which should be as hot as possible without scalding your hands. Because of the heat being generated there, a message is sent inside your body causing blood to shoot down to the hand area. By pulling the blood out of your head and into your hands, the pounding pressure of your migraine is relieved.

With migraines, Dr. Wiley insists that prevention is the key. A full 86 percent of headaches are unrelated to serious conditions. What this mean is that the majority of migraines can be prevented. By removing their triggers from our lives, we can easily live migraine-free.

Since dehydration is a main trigger, the simplest solution to prevent migraines is to stay hydrated throughout the day. It's estimated that most people are about two quarts short of their needed water intake each day, especially in the morning. Dr. Wiley suggests drinking two glasses of room-temperature water first thing in the morning to rehydrate from the sweating and breathing you've done overnight.

Another preventative measure you can take is to make sure you are on a solid sleep cycle. For migraine sufferers, it has been shown that the best sleep schedule is from ten o'clock in the evening to six o'clock in the morning. As mentioned previously, a good night's sleep will keep your serotonin levels up and allow your body to detox properly, fighting off migraines.

With a good night's sleep, you should be able to add a regular exercise routine to your schedule. This will keep your blood moving, increase your oxygen intake, and combat stress all in one fell swoop. A return to homeostasis is possible, and with it, a return to a migraine-free life under the Wellness Model of Health™.

Recommended Resources

Outwitting Headaches by Dr. Mark V. Wiley

The Live Pain Free Migraine Relief Kit

Learn more at www.endofalldiseases.com/migraineresources.

CHAPTER 17:

The End of Arthritis and Joint Pain

What Is Arthritis?

Many people wonder whether their chronic joint pain is arthritis or just a natural part of getting older. I want to be clear about one thing: most joint pain—regardless of the cause—is in fact arthritis.

I say this because, according to Dr. Mark Wiley in his best-selling book, *Arthritis Reversed*, arthritis is a term used to define a symptom, rather than a disease.

Dr. Wiley says that the majority of people with arthritis don't have actual arthritic diseases, such as juvenile or rheumatoid arthritis. Rather, they suffer from a series of symptoms that are classified as arthritis pain. For that reason, I'll use the term "arthritis" to refer to chronic joint pain in this chapter, whether you've seen a doctor and been "diagnosed" with arthritis or not.

In his research, Dr. Wiley learned that arthritis is believed to be the oldest discovered human ailment. Scientists have found this disease in the joints of some dinosaurs and even in mummies. He explains that the symptoms of arthritis are often universal and are largely experienced as stiffness, soreness, inflammation, and pain.

Over time, the cartilage between the joints can begin to wear down, exposing the joint to friction. When two bones rub together, inflammation and pain can take place. Redness and swelling of the joints and loss of joint function soon follow.

Arthritis includes more than one hundred different diseases or conditions that destroy joints, bones, muscles, cartilage, and other connective tissues, hampering or halting physical movement and causing pain. More than fifty million Americans have been diagnosed with some form of arthritis. And it's getting worse. Scientists project that by the year 2030, more than sixty-seven million Americans over the age of eighteen will be diagnosed with some form of arthritis.

But past, present, or future, one thing about arthritis remains constant: it has a debilitating impact on our simple, day-to-day activities, and it can keep us from living full, satisfying lives. The good news is that, as with the vast majority of ailments, it can be addressed from the ground up using the Wellness Model of Health™.

This chapter will discuss the misconceptions about arthritis. It will also tell you the true underlying causes of this condition, and what you can do to combat it.

The Myths and Lies of Arthritis

Arthritis is quite common and widespread, as are the myths and lies that surround it. It's important to distinguish what is true and what isn't so that you can find relief. Much of the information below comes from Dr. Mark Wiley, who was gracious enough to allow me to distill it for you in this chapter.

Arthritis Is a Part of Aging and Only Affects the Elderly

If you look around, it is easy to see how this myth formed and took hold. There are plenty of elderly people afflicted with arthritic conditions. And since many of the elderly show visible signs of arthritis (i.e., misshapen hands, walkers, and wheelchairs), one might conclude that it is a normal part of the aging process. However, this is not the case anymore.

By keeping the immune system strong and stable, eating right, exercising right, and taking care of bone and joint health, the onset and debilitating effects of arthritis need not be part of your aging process. And with better diagnosis and natural treatment remedies and therapies available, if you find you have the condition, you can stop it and reduce or even reverse its symptoms, so they will not progress into your senior years.

If You Have Arthritis, You Should Not Exercise

This is a myth most believed by those suffering the symptoms of arthritic pain and inflammation. Decades ago, patients were told not to exercise because it would rub the joints and make things worse. This is incorrect. While it is true that depending on your type of arthritis and other conditions, certain exercises should be avoided, this is not a blanket statement about all forms of exercise.

A certain amount of exercise can in fact greatly help reduce the symptoms of arthritis. Most often, those with arthritis in the hips and hands feel pain in the joints and inflammation and/or contraction in the muscles and tissues around those joints. However, part of what is contributing to the pain and stiffness is the limited range of motion within the joint structure that has happened as a result of not exercising.

The first step is to begin exercising slowly, lightly, and with limits, so as not to worsen or aggravate the conditions. Moving each joint slowly at first helps lubricate the joints and stretch the muscles. Strengthening exercises can help stabilize arthritic joint structures. This in turn helps bring fresh blood, and thus oxygen and nutrients, to the area, which decreases inflammation, stiffness, and pain. Then, as you are able, you can increase the time and rigor of your exercise.

Different Climates Have No Effect on Arthritis

The important issue here is that both cold and warm weather can affect arthritis in negative or positive ways. Climate does play a role in how you experience the symptoms of your condition.

Cold weather constricts muscles, tendons, and blood vessels, causing constriction around the joints, and thus pain and limited range of motion. Heat, on the other hand, allows muscles to expand and blood to flow, and so relieves compression around joints and helps move fresh blood into the arthritic area. This reduces pain and stiffness, and increases range of motion. Damp environments (whether warm or cold) cause inflammation around joints, and thus restrict movement and cause pain.

So while cold weather does not cause arthritis and warm weather does not cure it, it's clear that climate does play a role in how you experience your condition and its symptoms. This means that temperature and climate should not be ignored when putting an arthritis relief action plan into place.

Arthritis Sufferers Have to Live in Pain

This is a huge myth that is widely believed. Why? Because many arthritis sufferers do live in pain, with daily stiffness and inflammation. They are suffering greatly, yet needlessly, because they don't yet know all of the pieces of the puzzle that create homeostasis in our bodies. Once you are armed with this knowledge, you'll have the motivation and power to improve your health.

There are several methods for prevention and effective treatment that I will explain later in this chapter. Will there be a certain level of pain associated with your arthritis, even after mindfully doing all of the steps and taking all of the advice in this chapter? Perhaps. But it should be nowhere near the levels you feel today.

True Causes of Arthritis

Since true recovery means correcting the underlying cause rather than merely managing symptoms, we must first have at least a basic understanding of why our joints hurt.

Arthritis pain can almost always be traced back to some combination of these four primary causes: cartilage breakdown, bone degeneration, excess scar tissue, and muscle imbalances.

Even in cases of direct trauma or a damaging autoimmune disorder like rheumatoid arthritis, corrective action for one or more of these root causes can help your joint pain.

Cartilage Breakdown

Over time, your joint cartilage breaks down through sheer stress of use. That's normal. What's not normal is your body failing to repair and replace worn cartilage and leaving remnants of broken cartilage inside your joint—leaving you in pain.

If you participate in extreme sports, are overweight, or place your joints under other undue stress like repetitive, limited-range motion, your cartilage will break down even faster. This makes implementing the recovery strategies in this guide even more important if you wish to remain active and pain free.

So what prevents your joints from rebuilding?

First, inadequate hydration. As we've learned, well over half of your body is composed of water. As little as a 2 percent deficit can result in fatigue, reduced blood flow, and increased oxidative stress. Your body also needs enough fluids to flush away toxins. When dehydrated, toxin buildup can lead to painful trigger points and interfere with the healing process.

The second factor here is inadequate nutrition. As we covered in a previous chapter, most foods are grown in soil largely depleted of the key nutrients your body needs. Likewise, animals raised for food purposes are typically fed an unnatural diet, which affects the nutritional profile of the meat you eat. Without proper nutrition, our joints are unable to repair themselves.

Bone Degeneration

The second primary cause of arthritis is nearby bone degeneration. Yet the two main contributors to bone weakness may surprise you.

In the first place, you're far more likely to have a mineral imbalance than a calcium deficiency. Many foods have supplemental calcium and you may take additional calcium supplements, too. But your bones are made of many minerals, not just calcium.

As with cartilage breakdown, lacking the right balance of essential minerals can lead to bone degeneration. Again, increasing your calcium intake without maintaining a proper balance of other key nutrients is a recipe for painful bone spurs and bone weakness.

The other major contributor to bone weakness is lack of stimulation. Like muscle strength, bone strength is a matter of "use it or lose it." Inactivity leads to both lower bone density and decreased muscle strength, making you more likely to suffer injury and pain.

Joint Restriction

The third primary cause of joint pain is joint restriction. When your joint is restricted from moving smoothly, the resulting friction creates pain.

Whenever your body is injured, scar tissue is formed to seal and repair the damage. This is the scar tissue you see when your skin heals from a cut. But this also occurs internally.

However, your body's ability to shut down the inflammation and healing process decreases as you age. Over time, recovery from any injury takes longer than it used to. It's why you might twist your ankle as a child and be out bounding around the yard again in hours while the same injury may leave a senior citizen hobbled for weeks.

Underlying this age-related problem is a reduction in the body's production of systemic proteolytic enzymes. These enzymes are what tell your body to turn off the fires of inflammation when healing is complete. Then they help break down and carry away waste like the excess fibrin used to create scar tissue.

Without adequate levels of systemic proteolytic enzymes, even a minor injury like a twisted ankle or knee can lead to excess fibrin buildup. This creates an overgrown web of scar tissue, causing painful friction and restricted movement in the joint. Excess fibrin also clogs your arteries, hampering the blood flow that brings the oxygen and nutrients needed to repair the injury.

Muscle Imbalances

Muscle imbalances are one of the biggest causes of arthritis.

I discussed this topic in detail in chapter 7. In a nutshell, a muscle imbalance is formed when one muscle or a set of muscles is overused compared to an opposing muscle or set of muscles. The stronger muscles then pull the opposing muscles, along with nearby bones and joints, out of their normal positions. Once out of position, the joints are worn unevenly, leading to the breakdown and pain of arthritis.

When dealing with muscle imbalances, weight matters. Every pound of extra weight is equivalent to three pounds of compressive force on your joints. Since muscle imbalances pull your body off-center, carrying an extra ten pounds is like adding a thirty-pound weight to your already stressed joint.

The Mind Component

This final primary cause of joint pain may surprise you, but the mental component of pain cannot be overemphasized. Stress, emotions, and expectations all play a critical role in your pain and recovery, as I discussed in earlier chapters.

Persistent stress causes stress hormones like cortisol to soar, contributing to health issues throughout your body such as heart disease, increased fat build-up around your midsection, and widespread inflammation throughout your body—including painful joint inflammation.

Stress and negative emotions cause the muscles to tighten, constricting blood vessels. These tight muscles increase compressive pressure on your joints, while decreased blood circulation allows toxins to build up and inhibit the flow of oxygen and nutrients needed to repair damaged cartilage and bone. The outcome of this is restricted motion and pain.

Aside from the physical effects of stress, your own expectations directly influence your ability to recover. If you believe you will get better, you likely will. But the opposite is just as true; if you believe you won't get better, you likely won't.

Effective Treatment and Prevention for Arthritis

True recovery requires treating the root causes of your joint pain. Finding these causes will be a matter of exploration and discovery, and chances are you'll need to take two, three, or more of the approaches discussed here to get complete relief, because different solutions address different causes.

In this section, I'll start with the most basic steps everyone with joint pain should consider first.

Drink More Water

Replace at least some of your inflammatory sugary drinks like soda with water. Drink at least eight glasses of water each day—or more if you need it, due to a high activity level or other factors.

Dehydration really is one of the big, overlooked causes of joint pain. Moving on to the rest of these joint pain solutions before taking care of hydration would be a major mistake. Drink more water!

Replace Inflammatory Foods

Joint pain is usually a symptom of joint inflammation. And if you eat the standard Western diet, the very foods you eat are contributing to your pain.

Poor food choices will make your pain worse. Eat less (or preferably none) of the acidic, inflammatory foods listed in table 17.1—originally found in Dr. Wiley's book—for one week. Replace them with the more alkaline, anti-inflammatory options listed and notice the difference.

Table 17.1

EAT LESS OF THESE
Animal milk products (milk, cream, ice cream, cheese, cottage cheese, yogurt)
Hydrogenated oils (non-dairy creamer, crackers, cookies, chips, snack bars)
Nitrates (hot dogs, cold cuts, pepperoni, sausage, bacon, liverwurst)
Processed sugars (candy, soda, bread, bottled fruit juice, cookies, snack bars)
Nightshades (potatoes, peppers, tomatoes, eggplant, paprika)
Convenience and fast foods (french fries, onion rings, loaded baked potatoes, fatty burgers, Mexican food, pizza, calzones, stromboli)
Processed white flour products (flour, bread, pasta, pizza, crackers, preteens, donuts)
Animal milk products (milk, cream, ice cream, cheese, cottage cheese, yogurt)
Hydrogenated oils (non-dairy creamer, crackers, cookies, chips, snack bars)
Nitrates (hot dogs, cold cuts, pepperoni, sausage, bacon, liverwurst)
Processed sugars (candy, soda, bread, bottled fruit juice, cookies, snack bars)
Nightshades (potatoes, peppers, tomatoes, eggplant, paprika)
Convenience and fast foods (french fries, onion rings, loaded baked potatoes, fatty burgers, Mexican food, pizza, calzones, stromboli)
Processed white flour products (flour, bread, pasta, pizza, crackers, preteens, donuts)

EAT MORE OF THESE
Wild Alaskan salmon
Fresh whole fruits
Bright colored vegetables (except nightshades)
Green and white tea
Purified and distilled water
Healthy oils (olive, flax, hemp, safflower, hazelnut, coconut)
Certified organic beef and poultry
Nuts, legumes, and seeds
Dark green leafy vegetables
Organic oatmeal (regular, not instant)
Aromatic spices (turmeric, ginger, cloves, garlic, onion, coriander, ground mustard seed)

Correct Mineral Levels

While taking a quality vitamin and mineral supplement is a good idea, there's also a risk you're getting an excess of some minerals and a deficiency of others. As I discussed in great detail in chapter 14, proper nutrition requires a correct balance of key minerals.

Earlier, I covered the surprising fact that, for many concerned about bone strength, supplementing with too much calcium can be worse than not supplementing at all. Although your body requires calcium for strong bones, an excess of calcium in your system can signal your body to stop using it to strengthen your bones, or to use that excess to create painful bone spurs.

Remember, your bones are made of many minerals, not just calcium. The only way to know for sure which minerals your body needs is to have your mineral levels tested as a baseline. This is best performed before starting any new vitamin and mineral supplements. Your doctor or an independent lab can check your mineral levels using a simple hair analysis or blood work. Then supplement with the vitamins and minerals your body needs.

Exercise and Increased Activity

Fear of injury leads many joint pain sufferers to lead an inactive life. However, your bones and muscles require regular stimulation to remain strong. Inactivity puts you at more risk of injury, not less.

Consider introducing a regular exercise routine into your day. Below are brief descriptions of some exercises from Dr. Wiley's *Arthritis Reversed* you can incorporate into your routine to offer you some relief.

Mindful walking
Start slow by walking for twenty minutes a day. This will get the heart, lungs, muscles, and joints moving. This low-impact activity will keep you in balance, increase heart and lung function and blood and oxygen flow, burn off blood sugars and fats, and remove toxins and wastes through sweat.

QiGong standing pole exercises
QiGong is a system of exercising the body and internal organs to stretch, open the energy lines, release tension, clear the mind, balance respiration, and improve the circulation of energy, blood, and body fluids.

QiGong standing pole postures are a great way to begin exercising the body and connecting your body with your mind. In times when you are in too much pain to exercise or even walk, the standing pole exercises will help you to rehabilitate yourself and start feeling better, and can be a jumping-off point for next-level exercises.

Tai Chi
Tai Chi helps develop balance and prevent falls and fractures common in those with arthritis. It also helps build bone density and keeps muscles toned, while reducing stress by clearing the mind and regulating the heart and lungs. Through tai chi, you can also burn calories without taxing the joints. Additionally, it helps restore range of motion.

Yoga

Yoga is an ancient Indian practice of health and well-being that involves holding and moving between various postures, specified breathing methods, and achieving altered states of consciousness through meditation.

With extended practice of yoga, a level of fitness is achieved and weight loss experienced, which in turn further lower blood pressure and reduce the effects of daily stress. This reduction of stress, lowering of blood pressure, increased calmness of mind, and slowed breathing that yoga fosters are all useful tools in helping to reduce pain, along with the other symptoms and negative effects of arthritis.

Bodywork Therapies

Bodywork therapies are those that utilize the hands of a practitioner on your body to effect change in a positive way. Sometimes the hands-on approach is physical (like with massage) and breaks up connective tissue and relieves trigger points. At other times, the therapy may be interior via injection (such as in Prolozone™ therapy). In each case, you are relying on the healing hands of a trained practitioner to help correct imbalances in your body.

Many who suffer with arthritis find it difficult to exercise because they are either too weak, in too much pain, or have lost too much range of motion. In such cases, attending a series of hands-on bodywork sessions can really help loosen the body, align the system, free the nerves, and awaken the energy.

Energy Medicine

Energy medicine is another effective form of treatment for joint pain. I explored this concept in full in chapter 10 of this book.

The Mental Component

Mental stress and a negative outlook can sabotage your best efforts at beating joint pain.

Just as negative thoughts can keep you in pain, changing your mindset to a positive outlook can help you make dramatic improvements almost overnight. Best of all, there are numerous proven ways to do so without resorting to mind-numbing antidepressants and other pharmaceuticals.

Here are some of natural ways to boost your spirit and eliminate the negative mental blocks that may be keeping you in pain: adequate sleep, light therapy, meditation and hypnosis, binaural beats and brainwave training, the Sedona Method, and the Emotional Freedom Technique (EFT). For more on these methods, see the Recommended Resources section at the end of the chapter.

Supplements

You can mask joint pain with drugs, and continue to suffer. Or you can give your body the building blocks it needs to repair joint damage, strengthen weak bones, and stop the runaway inflammation that's causing your pain in the first place. That's the role these supplements play in your health.

In each of these supplements, potency matters. Look for good manufacturing control to ensure the supplement's ingredients are delivered in the correct particle size at the stated (preferably high) dose, so your body can absorb and use the ingredient in sufficient quantity to make a difference. I discussed supplements in detail in chapter 14.

Finally, these specific supplements are recommended because they're generally safer than many vitamins and minerals, with minimal or no side effects even when taken in high doses over time.

Topical Creams, Gels, and Oils

When searching for relief from pain, inflammation, swelling, and stiffness, many reach for some form of topical cream, gel, or ointment. Dr. Wiley points out that these products are found in abundance in American drugstores and Asian markets. Though the Eastern and Western versions of these products have some comparatively different ingredients, they serve the same purpose: instant relief for acute symptoms of arthritis.

Topical pain products are mostly used for short-term relief, as once their active ingredients have metabolized in the body, their value is greatly diminished. For effectiveness over the long term, they should be applied three times per day, and be part of an overall program for arthritis relief. On their own, these products can provide almost instant relief on some level to

Natural supplements for chronic joint pain:

- Avocado Soybean Unsaponifiables (ASU): slows down production of inflammatory chemicals in the body
- Boswellia Serrata: provides anti-inflammatory activity in areas of chronic inflammation
- Burdock Root: purifies blood and clears congestion from the circulatory, lymphatic, respiratory, and urinary system.
- Cetyl Myristoleate: promotes healthy joint function
- Chondroitin Sulfate: slows down joint cartilage breakdown
- Citrus Bioflavonoids: inhibits breakdown of connective tissue
- Devils Claw: has powerful NSAID-like properties
- Fish Oil/Omega-3 Fatty Acids: relieves pain and stiffness
- Glucosamine Sulfate: supports joint mobility and pain relief
- Hydrolyzed Collagen Type 2: lubricates the joints
- Ionic Minerals: helps cells absorb nutrients
- L-glutathione: strengthens the immune system
- Methylsulfonylmethane: improves cell permeability
- Paractin: helps correct imbalanced immune system
- Proteolytic Enzymes: helps control systemic inflammation
- Rutin: powerful antioxidant
- SAMe: relieves pain
- Thunder God Vine: regulates the immune system and reduces inflammation
- White Willow Bark: reduces inflammation and pain
- Vitamins: aids in growth, repair, bone density, pH balance, and hormone regulation

one or more symptoms and can be used to help you get through your day or night.

When shopping for a topical pain product, be sure to look for items that are made with few unnatural ingredients, and that include the following:

- Camphor oil: calms nerve pain, reduces inflammation, and is used as an anesthetic, disinfectant, and sedative

- Capsaicin: diminishes the chemical in the body known as substance P, which is involved in transmitting pain signals to the brain

- Menthol: numbs, expands blood vessels, cools the heat of inflammation

- Wintergreen: a counterirritant

Be sure to use these treatments carefully and as directed.

Frequency Specific Microcurrent Therapy

Research has found that injured tissues in your body emit different electrical frequencies than healthy tissues. By counteracting the electrical frequencies emitted by injured tissue, you can get fast pain relief and as much as a three-fold reduction in healing time.

Frequency Specific Microcurrent (FSM) is a painless therapy that applies these counteracting frequencies to your body using extremely low power electric current through electrodes and conductive gloves.

FSM technology has been around for nearly a century, but was blocked by the traditional medical establishment for much of that time. It has only come into widespread use over the past fifteen years.

Prolozone™ Therapy

Prolozone™ combines concepts of neural therapy, prolotherapy, and ozone therapy into a single treatment that typically results in immediate pain relief and rapid healing of degenerated joints.

The key to its clinical success is the use of injected medical-quality ozone into the injured joint. Even healthy ligaments and joints typically get only one tenth of the oxygen of nearby tissue. Injured and inflamed joints get even less oxygen as circulation is further impaired—reducing oxygen utilization.

Your cells need oxygen to produce energy. But in situations where oxygen utilization is impaired, more oxygen is converted to free radical molecules—increasing the deterioration rate of your joint. Ozone has an unstable third oxygen atom, which when injected in your joint, can be utilized by cells to overcome this oxygen utilization deficit with dramatic results.

Prolozone™ also includes procaine for fast numbing pain relief, anti-inflammatory medicines, vitamins, minerals and proliferative agents, and so stimulates regeneration. While this therapy is slightly invasive with the injection and may not be 100 percent all natural depending on the anti-inflammatory and proliferative agents used, it has a highly safe track record and such an astounding impact on joints that I felt it necessary to share it here as an advanced joint pain solution.

You Have a Choice

Arthritis is one of the most common ailments out there, affecting nearly one in five Americans. It can be debilitating, but when you work from the Wellness Model of Health™, there are many steps you can take to find relief. Making the right choices in your diet and exercise, as well as having a positive mental attitude, can make the difference between resigning yourself to a life of pain and working toward a pain-free existence.

Recommended Resources

Comprehensive Information about Arthritis

Get a free copy of Dr. Mark Wiley's book, *Arthritis Reversed: Groundbreaking 30 Day Arthritis Relief Action Plan* for only the cost of shipping at http://www.losethebackpain.com/arthritisbook.php.

Effective, All Natural Joint Supplement

Protect and rebuild your joints using the most effective, all-natural joint supplement on the market, Super Joint Support™ at www.losethebackpain.com/superjointsupport.html.

CHAPTER 18:

The End of Chronic Back Pain

What Is Chronic Back Pain?

We often use the expression "pain in the neck" to describe someone who just won't go away.

For so many people, "pain in the back" would be more accurate. For those suffering from chronic back pain, persistent pain is a common experience. It might be constant, or it might come and go at the worst times. In either case, it's just not going away.

I literally wrote the book on chronic back pain, *The 7 Day Back Pain Cure*. Whether it's a dull lower back pain, or radiating upper back pain that moves to the arms and shoulders, one thing is for sure: chronic back pain can be debilitating and it can affect every area of your life, until you take your health into your own hands by following the Wellness Model of Health™. When your natural state of homeostasis moves back in, the chronic back pain moves out.

There are two major types of chronic back pain: lower and upper pain.

Lower Back Pain

People suffering from general lower-back pain usually complain of one of two types of discomfort. The first is a dull, aching feeling, a tight, "locked up" sensation that limits movement. The second is a sharp pain. Sometimes these sensations are accompanied by radiating pain in the legs and/or feet. All these symptoms can be caused by imbalances (a lack of homeostasis) within your physical body, mind (e.g., stress), and/or diet.

Upper Back Pain

If you're suffering from general upper back pain, you're probably having a hard time doing daily activities like driving a car, working at the computer, or even brushing your teeth. You may be experiencing headaches or radiated pain into the arms and/or the shoulder blades.

You may have had muscles "lock up," making it nearly impossible to move your head or arms. All these symptoms can also be caused by problems with your body (usually muscle trauma or imbalances), mind (e.g., stress), and/or diet—and most likely, they've been building up for quite some time.

This region of our back is quite complex due to the fact that it contains many joints. When working properly, you can perform everyday tasks with ease—but when pain strikes in the upper back, even the simplest activities can be difficult.

The Myths and Lies of Chronic Back Pain

In order to effectively put an end to chronic back pain, we first have look beyond the symptoms of the pain itself. Instead, we must turn our attention to figuring out and fixing the underlying problem causing the pain.

However, before I get to these causes, let's look at some of the most enduring and popular myths about back pain.

Myth #1: You "Throw Out" Your Back

Oftentimes, back pain is preceded by some physical activity, like picking up a heavy object, sneezing, or bending over. The usual thinking goes, "Well, since I didn't have back pain before doing this activity, the activity must have caused the back pain." The actual answer is usually much more complicated than that. True, physical activity can trigger a pain episode, but by itself, it isn't the underlying cause.

Myth #2: Back Pain Means There's Something Wrong with Your Back

It's understandable that many people would assume that, if they have back pain, then something must be wrong mechanically with their back. And indeed, this may be part of the problem, but it is rarely the sole cause of the problem.

Other factors often come into play, originating from the mind (i.e., stress or emotional distress) or from your diet (i.e., unhealthy foods) that can cause severe back pain episodes even when nothing is physically wrong with your spine, discs, joints, muscles, or ligaments. These factors can also exacerbate physical issues, making existing back pain worse.

Myth #3: My Current Back Pain Isn't Related to Previous Bouts

For most people, the trigger that causes their back pain episode is different on different occasions, which leads to the thinking that today's back pain has nothing to do with the back pain experienced two months ago. In fact, multiple back pain episodes are usually caused by the same underlying problem—even if the apparent trigger for different episodes appears to vary.

Myth #4: Being Overweight Is a Major Cause of Back Pain

While it's true that being overweight can contribute to back pain, in most instances, it's only a minor cause of this. Bottom line, our spines are designed to support the weight of the body, whether we're carrying around extra pounds or not. Being overweight can, though, create an extra burden for those who already have back problems, making it more difficult to move around and get exercise when pain strikes.

Myth #5: People Who Are Not Active Are More Likely to Have Back Pain

Because active people are believed to be stronger than those who are inactive, it's thought that active people are less likely to suffer from back pain. In fact, the opposite is true. Active people put themselves at higher risk of back pain because they place greater strain on their muscles and exert themselves more often. Back pain isn't caused by weakness; as we'll learn in the next section, it's caused by muscle imbalances, injuries, or illness.

Myth #6: The Best Thing for Back Pain Is Bed Rest

While severe back pain may constitute a need for limited mobility and bed rest, in the long run, prolonged bed rest can actually cause more pain and problems. Faster healing occurs when you take measures to treat the cause, including exercise and activities to increase your blood flow, range of motion, and flexibility. Too much time in bed can prolong your pain and healing time, and can also cause muscle attrition and weakness, which in turn makes your body more susceptible to injury.

Now that I've debunked some of the most common myths about back pain, let's take a closer look at what really causes it.

True Causes of Chronic Back Pain

Depending on the type of chronic back pain you are suffering from, the causes can vary. Some of the causes are easy to pinpoint, while others can be a consequence of an action that you aren't even aware of.

Lower Back Pain

Lower back pain can be caused by a number of different things. Ranking at the top of the list are pulled muscles, disc problems (herniated, bulging discs), arthritic conditions, or joint dysfunction. In addition, trigger points, pinched nerves, spinal compression, or torsion can be common causes, though many people don't recognize this connection. Still other causes can lie in stress and negative emotions, as I covered in earlier chapters. Trauma (injury) and muscle imbalances are the most common causes of lower back pain.

While you would know if a precise trauma caused your pain, you probably wouldn't be aware of a muscle imbalance until it resulted in pain. That's because it happens slowly over a period of time. Muscle imbalances affect your posture, causing "postural dysfunctions," which may include abnormal alignment of the pelvis and abnormal curvature of the spine.

This misalignment causes increased wear and tear on the joints, muscles, and ligaments—even the discs.

Upper Back Pain

The three most common reasons for upper back pain are trauma, trigger points, and muscle imbalances. With trauma, it's easy to determine what caused the pain; however, in case of trigger points or muscle imbalances, a person may not be able to pinpoint any one thing that triggered it. That's because postural dysfunctions, as referred to above, are often the culprit.

It's important to understand that while upper back pain caused by postural dysfunctions or muscle imbalance can introduce itself suddenly, it probably took a long time to develop before any pain was perceived. This is also true of trigger points, which can occur after toxins build up in tissues, muscles, tendons, or ligaments for a period of time.

All Back Pain

For some people, the cause of chronic back pain is not related to a traumatic injury. For these people, no matter what they try and no matter what type of practitioner they see for their pain, they still suffer. The problem could very well be psychosomatic, meaning the issue is related to both mind and body and how they interact.

Negative thought patterns, especially stress, can keep you from recovering and make your condition worse by amplifying the pain and other symptoms.

As I discussed in chapter 2, stress is an interesting phenomenon. It means different things to different people. What we each individually consider to be stressful is largely a matter of our perception. Our perceptions are our realities, and so what we think poses a threat actually does so by virtue of our established belief system. What's more, there are many kinds of stressors—physical (the response to being frightened), emotional (loss of a loved one), psychological (obsessive thoughts), spiritual (loss of faith), and psychosomatic (the need for attention).

The effect of such prolonged or recurring stress is that it keeps the autonomic nervous system from balancing, or achieving your natural state of homeostasis. Stress can also lead to depression, anxiety, muscle tension, insomnia, and body pain. All of these are known triggers of various mental and physical (mind/body) illnesses and diseases, including chronic back pain.

Effective Treatments and Prevention for Chronic Back Pain

Traditional treatments offered by physicians for chronic back pain include cortisone injections, muscle relaxants, or non-steroidal anti-inflammatory drugs. In some instances, surgery is suggested, but it should always be your last option.

Traditional treatment from chiropractors and physical therapists may include spinal mobilization, hot packs, ultrasound, electrical stimulation, and therapeutic exercises. Sometimes these can be helpful, but only when they are actually needed.

Note that I said "traditional treatments" above and not "effective treatments." In most cases, these treatments, while common, do not address the cause of the pain. Instead, they only mask or delay its recurrence. For example, if you need a spinal adjustment, a chiropractor can be very helpful. However, if your pain comes from trigger points, a spinal adjustment will not give you any relief. That's why it's so important to understand that the treatment has to address the cause of the pain. The cause should dictate where, how, and from whom you seek help.

As I covered in previous chapters, many causes of back pain come from muscle imbalances. Lower back pain caused by muscles imbalances cannot be treated effectively through most of the above treatments. In order to reduce or eliminate the pain, you first have to correct what caused it. The most effective treatment is to correct the muscle imbalance and restore postural balance. This treatment works in relieving lower back pain and in preventing future incidences of it.

The following action plan covers two areas: 1) short-term and temporary pain relief, and 2) long-term solutions.

For each category of pain relief (temporary versus long term), the solutions below have been arranged in order, with the step likely to help you the most listed first. Start with the solution at the top of the list, and then work your way down only if the pain improves but doesn't completely disappear.

Temporary Pain Relief—Action Plan

Temporary pain relief for chronic back pain can be obtained from quality pain-relief creams, natural anti-inflammatories, and far infrared heat therapy.

The same topical creams, gels, and oils used for arthritis, as discussed in chapter 17, can also be applied to ease chronic back pain. For suggestions on natural anti-inflammatory supplements, see chapter 14 for more information.

Far infrared heat therapy is another excellent option for temporary pain relief. If you ever reach for a heating pad to try to relax and soothe painful and tight muscles, then you're already familiar with standard heat therapy. However, few people experience true relief from a regular heating pad. This is because typical heating pads simply warm the skin. They don't penetrate into the tissues and muscles where your pain thrives, and that's why they rarely give you lasting relief.

Far infrared heat therapy solves that problem by sinking deep into your tissues for longer-lasting, healing relief. Think of how good it feels to soak in the sun—that delicious, bone-deep warmth you feel from its rays. That feeling comes from the sun's infrared rays. Infrared waves are different from the ultraviolet waves that can contribute to sunburn. They don't harm your skin and they make your muscles feel great. You can't see them, because they have a longer wavelength than visible light, but you can feel them.

Infrared light that is farthest from visible light is called "far infrared," and it has been used to promote healing for years. For example, a 2010 study by the Department of Rehabilitation and Physical Medicine of patients with chronic fatigue syndrome found that participants experienced considerable relief from symptoms with daily far infrared treatment. Numerous other studies have also found that far infrared heat helps everything from burning fat effectively to killing cancer cells.

Regular (non-infrared) heating pads use high-temperature heat to attempt to deliver heat deep into your muscles, but those near-burning temperatures cause too much pain for most people. In comparison, far infrared heating pads use moderate-temperature heat at a particular wavelength (the far infrared wavelength) that penetrates deeply into your muscles naturally.

Again, that deep penetration is the reason far infrared heat is so effective at soothing pain, relaxing muscles, improving circulation, and reducing fatigue. Just like those invisible sun rays, far infrared heat has been shown in scientific studies to actually sink two to three inches into muscles and ligaments. As it does this, it transforms light energy into heat energy, expanding blood vessels, improving circulation, and encouraging the healing process.

And that's only the beginning. There are even more health benefits to far infrared heat. As blood circulation improves, toxins break down and flush out of the body. Things like uric acid, sodium, metals, and fat-soluble toxins all vacate the muscles and tissues, freeing the body to heal itself with its own strength and abilities.

Blood pressure decreases, muscle cramps relax, oxygen transport increases, and fatigue melts away. Even better, because the heat goes so deep into the tissues, these beneficial effects can last for up to six hours, depending on how long you soak in the heat.

So how do you take advantage of this deep-penetrating pain reliever? There are several far infrared devices out there, from small pads to four-person saunas. You can learn more about far infrared therapy and see which devices I recommend at www.losethebackpain.com/heat.

Long-Term Relief—Action Plan

Long-term relief for chronic back pain should be a combination of the following: muscle-balance therapy, trigger-point therapy, inversion therapy, emotional troubleshooting, and dietary adjustments.

Most of you will experience welcome relief using the first five long-term relief steps described below. You'll probably be surprised at how quickly your pain goes away. But for those few who have battled with back pain for a long time, the "layered" approach may be the only way to go.

This is usually because your back pain is caused by a multitude of factors and perhaps has become so "normal" for your body that it will take a longer, more comprehensive approach to break the cycle.

The key is to use the treatments suggested, in the order suggested, and at the same time until you can figure out the right combination that works for you. Once you have this figured out, you can stop using the treatments that you suspect aren't as effective, thereby arriving at the simplest possible solution.

Step 1: Hydrate

I have already covered the importance of water and adequate hydration in past chapters. It should go without saying that one of the most important things you can do for your health is to drink more water.

Earlier, I mentioned how the discs in your spine are made up mostly of water. When you drink more, you re-inflate those discs, which have probably been depleted of fluids throughout the day. Water helps eliminate toxins from your body, and constant cleansing can prevent trigger points from forming and reduce the severity of any trigger points already present in the muscle tissues.

Drinking water helps joints function more smoothly, because it cushions the muscles and provides more support for the body's movement. It also fills the stomach, which can deter us from eating too much, and helps to keep our energy levels high.

Step 2: Reduce Stress and Negative Emotions

If you've used the combination of muscle-balance therapy, trigger point therapy, and inversion therapy for several weeks and you're still experiencing pain, it may be time to evaluate your emotional state of mind.

The following recommendations for reducing stress are taken from Dr. Mark Wiley's book, *Arthritis Reversed*.

Tips for stress busting:
1. Walk outside for at least twenty continuous minutes every day.
2. Quiet the mind and calm the nerves with meditation.
3. Take ten deep belly breaths every hour.
4. Drink plenty of pure water.
5. Avoid sugar in all forms and limit caffeine.
6. Regulate sleep and wake cycles to a consistent daily routine.
7. Prioritize your life, work, family, and personal time and activities.
8. Do six shoulder shrugs whenever you are tense.
9. Realize that when people criticize and judge, they are labeling an "image" of you and not you personally.
10. Realize that you are worth so much more than the sum of your titles, money, and belongings.

In most cases, if someone is not feeling a lot better by the time they've adopted these three therapies—particularly if the person is doing them diligently on a daily basis—the problem is often a case of severe stress and, in some extreme cases, lingering anger from some emotional trauma (e.g., divorce, abuse, abandonment).

More often than not, the stresses are job pressures, relationship issues, health concerns (if the person is dealing with a serious disease or troubling diagnosis), significant losses, career confusion, or family troubles.

Evaluate the stresses in your life and see if you can reduce some of them. If you suspect an old trauma may be affecting you, consider an appointment with a licensed therapist. At the very least, carve out some personal time to reflect and record your thoughts, talk to a trusted friend, or purchase some helpful books—anything that might help you get to the core of your pain.

Step 3: Muscle-Balance Therapy

As I talked about earlier, muscle-balance therapy is an approach that works for everyone—regardless of the condition your doctor may have diagnosed—because we all have muscle imbalances.

For many people, muscle-balance therapy is all that's needed. For others, additional treatments may be necessary. As mentioned earlier, very rarely is chronic back pain caused by one thing; instead, it's often the result of a combination of causes. Therefore, your treatment plan should include a combination of treatments.

Muscle-balance therapy is an innovative approach to eliminating back pain (and just about any other ailment) by addressing the imbalances in your muscles. In essence, it attempts to reverse the process that created the pain in the first place and bring your body back to a more neutral, properly aligned or "balanced" state.

The muscle-balance therapy approach begins by assessing the strength and flexibility of your muscle pairs—in your hips, pelvis, spine, and throughout the body. The idea is to find out which muscles are strong and which are weak, which are tight and which are more flexible, and which may be overworked or shortened.

Since these various imbalances stress joints, other muscles, and ligaments, the goal of the therapy is to rebalance the muscles so that each muscle pair is as close to "normal" as possible. By evening out the muscle tension between the left and right sides of the body or between the front and back, the body supports the spine more evenly, automatically improving posture, allowing vertebrae to move back into position, and taking pressure off irritated nerves and muscles—thereby eliminating chronic back pain.

Step 4: Trigger Point Therapy

After one to two weeks of using muscle-balance therapy, if you're still experiencing pain, it's time to add trigger point therapy to your routine.

Trigger point therapy can help eliminate muscle pain and spasms that muscle-balance therapy may not have been able to address. However, don't stop the muscle-balance therapy, as it does many things for you that trigger point therapy can't. These benefits include strengthening weak muscles, lengthening short and tight muscles, working to correct imbalances, and most importantly, eliminating the dysfunction.

Remember that trigger points can be persistent points of pain, and because of their position in the muscle fibers, they can keep you feeling stiff and sore.

For a detailed description of trigger point therapy, see Chapter 8.

Step 5: Spinal Decompression

After two weeks of combined muscle-balance therapy and trigger point therapy, if you still aren't completely pain free, it's time to add spinal decompression therapy to your routine.

I discussed this method in detail in chapter 9. Combining spinal decompression therapy with muscle-balance therapy is a very effective way to relieve all kinds of back pain. Often, when muscle-balance therapy and trigger point therapy aren't enough to get you to 100 percent, the problem is a disc that's still bulging enough to put pressure on a nerve somewhere in the spine.

Muscle-balance therapy rebalances the muscles so they no longer pull the spine out of alignment, but that alone may not be enough to allow the discs to "pop" back into place or provide enough of an increase in blood flow to promote healing. In other words, your muscles are probably closer to properly supporting your back, but the vertebrae may need some assistance in getting back to their ideal position, where they'll no longer impact the nerves.

This is where spinal decompression therapy can be extremely effective. Since the human body is upright most of the time, gravity is constantly placing downward pressure on the spine, which is referred to as "compression." Turning the body upside down allows gravity to pull the spine in the opposite direction, opening up the spaces between the vertebrae. This often encourages the discs to return to a healthy position and, if torn, to heal themselves.

Again, a few minutes a day of this therapy can be enough to help you start experiencing significant relief. And with literally millions of success stories, it's definitely something you'll want to consider.

Step 6: Dietary Adjustments

If you've gotten to this point and you're still experiencing pain, don't lose hope. Your diet could have a lot to do with it.

First, you should continue with the steps outlined above. Some people with particularly stubborn chronic back pain just need to hang in there a little longer to see results. Remember, your back pain took a long time to develop and it may just need more time to right itself—especially if you have a very stubborn case.

This is particularly true if you have a lot of causes contributing to the pain, such as muscle imbalances, trigger points, bulging discs, and emotional stressors. And don't be surprised if that's the case, as it's actually very common to have numerous causes, some of which require a lot of digging to uncover.

Continue with the previous steps and, in addition, start adjusting your diet. Though diet usually doesn't cause back pain all by itself, it can certainly make existing back pain worse or create conditions in the body that make it harder to heal. Sometimes, diet is what pushes your pain level "over the edge" to the point where you can really feel it.

You may be eating a lot of things that could be increasing the inflammation in your muscles and nerves. If you're overweight, the extra pounds could be making it more difficult to rebalance your muscles. Your diet also could be increasing the toxins in your system, contributing to trigger points.

While I discussed inflammatory foods at length in chapter 12, it's worth covering them here again in brief. Here are seven categories of foods that should be avoided if you're experiencing severe pain and inflammation:

1. Animal milk products

2. Hydrogenated oils

3. Nitrates

4. Processed sugars

5. Nightshades

6. Convenience foods

7. Processed white flour products

Are you surprised? As you can see, most of the items on this list are actually the staple American diet. Is it any wonder Americans are among the most obese and pain suffering peoples in the world?

Even if you're doing trigger point therapy every night, if you're still eating foods like the ones listed above that put more toxins back into your body during the day, you'll just be maintaining your current condition rather than improving it. Likewise, you may not be drinking enough water, which could be depriving your discs of the shock absorption they need or contributing to toxic buildup in your muscles.

Changing your diet could be the one thing you need to tip the scales in favor of your recovery. Your body needs good, wholesome food to give it the strength and power it needs to heal. And just like with emotional changes, you can implement dietary changes at the very beginning of your treatment program and continue choosing more healthful foods as you work on the physical treatments.

Additional Treatment Options

There are various additional treatments you can try to eliminate your chronic back pain. As I mentioned earlier, a layered approach often works best. It is important to note, however, that none of these should be tried until after you've worked your way through the six steps we just covered.

Frequency Specific Microcurrent therapy

In combination with a proper diagnosis, Frequency Specific Microcurrent (FSM) therapy delivers currents to the afflicted area, sending energy that renews cells and reduces pain. FSM works on biophysics principles, actually altering or changing tissue and reducing inflammation and scarring. Some find immediate relief upon the first treatment, and over time, the pain is eliminated altogether.

FSM is usually delivered in a series of treatments performed on a regular basis. After the desired pain relief has been achieved, the patient can be prescribed a home unit where they can continue self-treatment if necessary.

Of those who have tried FSM therapy, some have received relief—others have not. One good thing about the treatment is that even if it doesn't help, it doesn't hurt. So there is relatively little or no danger or any risky side effects to FSM therapy.

Stem cell treatment

Another treatment alternative for those suffering with chronic back pain from degenerated, damaged, or herniated intervertebral discs uses stem cells to regenerate the discs. This option does more than remove the pain—it also cures the problem that caused it.

An alternative to risky back surgery, stem cell regeneration was developed in the United Kingdom by Dr. Stephen Richardson. A relatively new procedure, it was discovered in 2006. Among its many benefits is the fact that the body cannot reject the stem cells, because they come from the patient, not a donor.

How does it work? The patient's own mesenchyme stem cells (MSC) are combined with a collagen gel that is surgically implanted into the area. It's safer and less invasive than traditional back surgery and has fewer side effects.

This stem cell treatment does what your body would optimally do on its own, if conditions were right. Those conditions include drinking plenty of water, maintaining a healthy diet with the proper amount of vitamins and minerals, and avoiding stress and negativity.

Prolozone™ therapy

Dr. Frank Shallenberger pioneered Prolozone™ therapy, a technique that injects oxygen into damaged tissues, joints, ligaments, and tendons. As discussed previously, this technique is based on the circulation of blood throughout the body, which transports vitamins, minerals, and oxygen. Low levels of oxygen can create pain. When oxygen is reintroduced into those areas, healing begins.

Prolozone™ involves three specific techniques. Injected first are homeopathic anti-inflammatory medications, which reduce inflammation and swelling, thus increasing circulation in the area. Then, specific vitamins and minerals are added to promote healing. The last step is injecting ozone into the afflicted area. The average person needs three to five treatments.

Prolozone™ has seen success in treating musculoskeletal and joint pain, including chronic neck and back pain, degenerated discs, and shoulder pain, as well as other pain not related to the back or neck. Its effects have been permanent for some—because it corrects what causes the pain in the first place. Those with chronic back pain have a 75 percent chance of being pain free forever.

It's Not a Life Sentence

If you suffer from chronic back pain, chances are you don't even remember what life was like before your pain. You probably find that things you do in your day-to-day life bring you pain that prevents you from accomplishing tasks and even finding joy.

Remember, no matter how you feel right now, chronic back pain is not a life sentence. Using the Complete Healing Formula™, you have the power to bring balance back to the way you handle emotions like stress, coupled with the short-term and long-term solutions discussed here. You have the power to return your back to a state of natural homeostasis. And that could be the key to you getting your life back.

Recommended Resources

Dr. Stephen Richardson

To learn more about stem cell therapy and Dr. Richardson's work, visit www. losethebackpain.com/stemcells.

Ozone Practitioners List

Dr. Frank Shallenberger, the creator of Prolozone™ Therapy, trains doctors in the use of Prolozone™ and other related ozone therapies. You can find a local doctor trained in the medical use of ozone on this list www.oxygenhea1ingtherapies.com/my ozone doctor.com.html.

Muscle Imbalances

To learn more about muscle imbalances and how to address them to eliminate back pain, visit www.losethebackpain.com/getstarted.hml.

Far Infrared Heat

To learn about the healing powers of far infrared heat, and how you can benefit from them, visit www.losethebackpain.com/heat.

The 7-Day Back Pain Cure

For the most comprehensive book on eliminating back pain, request a free copy of my book, *The 7-Day Back Pain Cure* at www.losethebackpain. com/7daybackpaincure.html.

The Lose the Back Pain® System™

Identify pain-causing muscle imbalances and use the excrcise routines included in The Healthy Back Institute's *Lose the Back Pain® System™* to eliminate imbalances in your body. To get started, visit www.losethebackpain. com/getstarted.html.

CHAPTER 19:

The End of Osteoporosis

What Is Osteoporosis?

Admit it: the first thing you think about when you hear the word "osteoporosis" is milk.

But, as I covered earlier, this is a flawed assumption. The truth is that milk is only good for you if you're a baby cow. Not only does drinking milk not help with osteoporosis, it actually causes inflammation and pain. To make matters worse, when the milk comes from sick, factory-raised cows, filled with antibiotics and hormones, it can be even more harmful.

Osteoporosis is a condition that decreases the density and quality of our bones, increasing the risk for fracture. And it affects a huge number of people.

According to the International Osteoporosis Foundation, the numbers surrounding osteoporosis are staggering. Estimated to affect two hundred million women worldwide, and resulting in more than 8.9 million annual bone fractures, this ailment is one of the most prevalent causes of pain and suffering on the world stage today.

And these figures are just for women. In the US alone, the National Osteoporosis Foundation counts forty-four million more people who either have osteoporosis or are at high risk for it due to low bone density. Furthermore, projections suggest that by 2020, half of all Americans over the age of fifty will show signs of low bone density.

The Wellness Model of Health™ hold the keys to stopping and even reversing osteoporosis. In this chapter, I'll cover the truths and untruths about osteoporosis, as well as the actions you can take to combat this disease at its source.

The Myths and Lies of Osteoporosis

It's a common general misconception that drinking milk will prevent you from getting osteoporosis and possibly even reverse its effects. I covered this myth briefly when sharing Dr. Thompson's work on minerals and *The Calcium Lie*.

In addition, Vivian Goldschmidt, MA, has studied osteoporosis extensively, and she says that if a calcium deficiency was the cause of osteoporosis, then it would cease to exist. All anyone would need to do is take calcium supplements, which she says is clearly not the solution.

I spoke to Goldschmidt in an interview for my *Live Pain Free* newsletter. According to her, another myth about this ailment is that drugs are necessary to cure osteoporosis. The reality is that this is far from the case. The drugs actually create a greater imbalance, which in turn creates a vicious cycle of drugs and doctor visits, pushing you further and further away from a state of homeostasis and true health.

The mainstream media ignores the true causes of osteoporosis because, if sufferers knew the truth, they would realize that they don't need the drugs. And as I discussed before, pharmaceuticals are a multi-million dollar industry.

Nearly all health conditions are typically treated with a drug, but it is not a deficiency of the drug in your body that is causing the problem. The real problem is biochemical imbalance, which I will explore later in this chapter.

The True Causes of Osteoporosis

You've heard it before: "You are what you eat." In Goldschmidt's *Save Our Bones* program, she says that modern diseases are caused by modern diets. People just aren't eating the way that they should be.

I covered the dietary implications of mineral deficiency earlier in this book, but a key fact bears repeating. Bones are a critical storehouse for at least twelve of the body's critical minerals. Our bodies rely on our bones to store and release particular minerals to perform different functions.

When we fuel the body with the nutrients and minerals it needs, our bones have an ample supply of minerals to keep up with the body's needs. Almost like a checking account, as long as we're depositing enough minerals to keep up with what we spend, all remains well.

However, deficiencies in our modern diet force our bones to bear the weight of our nutritional problems. Rather than keeping an even flow of input and output, our bones give more minerals to the body's functions than they are able to accumulate. Over time, this depletes the bones of their minerals—just like an overdrawn checking account.

Beyond mineral intake alone, a little knowledge of the body's chemistry brings an even greater truth to light about osteoporosis: the role of pH balance. The pH balance in your blood should be at a certain level to keep you healthy. But our modern diets, stress levels, and environments are wreaking havoc on the body's the pH level, which leads to a biochemical imbalance.

What does this have to do with osteoporosis? When our pH level swings out of balance—usually by becoming too acidic—the body reacts to correct this balance. In the case of too much acidity, the body looks for ways to restore balance using alkalizing agents. Calcium is one of the body's most high-powered alkalizing agents, and it is therefore drained out of our bones in the body's attempt to alkalize our acidic blood levels.

Nutrition is not the only culprit when it comes to your pH level. When it comes to too much acidity in our bodies, stress—which you will now recognize as a running theme in this book—strikes again. Stress causes the body to release acidic cortisol. The chronic state of stress leads to a continued buildup of cortisol in the bloodstream, which has an acidifying effect in our bodies.

Toxins can also affect your pH level. And we're not just talking about the toxins you ingest, but also the ones that you put on your skin. There are creams full of chemicals that people slather on their skin—the largest organ in the body. These toxins are quickly absorbed into your bloodstream, where they have an acidifying effect.

Your environment could also be toxic. Paints, new cars, mattresses, and chemical stain-resistant sprays on furniture can all be highly toxic. Chlorinated water is another offender. And these are things you come into contact with every day. Each of these toxins does further damage to your body's pH balance, driving the acidity to an even higher level.

Goldschmidt's work explores pH levels at length as a key factor in bone health. She explains that once your pH level is acidified, your body does everything it can to rebalance it to a more alkaline level—including leaching calcium from your bones, as I explained. While the body does hold reserves of alkalizing agents to keep up with occasional acidic foods, these reserves are insufficient to sustain extended periods of acidity. Without making changes, your alkaline reserves can be depleted over time.

As I mentioned, to correct an excess of acidity in the blood, the bones will release alkaline calcium, depleting their calcium stores. Although calcium is only one of the minerals critical to bone strength, expending it to correct the blood's pH level has a compounding effect over time. Goldschmidt notes that your body will make any sacrifice to restore your pH level—even at the cost of its own structural integrity.

Effective Treatment and Prevention for Osteoporosis

Now you know how acidic foods affect your bones. So how should you adjust your diet?

Calcium supplementation is often the first question that comes up when we talk about osteoporosis. But as I discussed before, and as Dr. Robert Thompson reveals in his books, *The Calcium Lie* and *The Calcium Lie II*, increased calcium supplementation is actually linked to increases in bone fractures. Not only does an excess of calcium in the diet cause various heart and health problems, it doesn't even effectively address bone strength.

Instead of blindly taking calcium supplements, Dr. Thompson reports that trace minerals—like those found in sea salt—are helpful when it comes to stopping and reversing the loss of bone density. These mineral supplements do include calcium, but in a proper balance with other minerals. Additionally, a mineral analysis will reveal what foods you should add or remove from your diet to find a proper balance of minerals, which will take you a long way toward true homeostasis and recovery.

The key to preventing and reversing osteoporosis resides in a balanced diet. To be clear, I'm not talking about the balanced diet we all learned in school, with the USDA's ever-changing groups of food plates and food pyramids. I'm referring to managing the excesses and deficiencies in our diets, so that we can maintain a healthy, balanced pH level in our bodies.

Goldschmidt outlines a clear path to addressing osteoporosis in her *Save Our Bones* program. A pH-friendly diet isn't a situation where you should never eat one thing or always eat another. The goal is to balance out your diet so that your alkaline reserves never get depleted.

We're all called to understand how to eat for ourselves, rather than getting a list from someone else of what to eat and when. In this way, we learn to make simple decisions on our own, which makes such lifestyle changes easier for us to sustain. By now, you know a lot about acidic and alkalizing foods from the chapters on arthritis and chronic back pain. This is a great place to put that knowledge to work.

Once people take control of their food choices, they start to feel better and more energized. And when they do go to eat something unhealthy, like a Twinkie for example, their bodies tell them right away that it is not a good food to eat. In short, the guidelines for eating when it comes to osteoporosis can have added benefits for your overall health.

Once you've found a balanced diet, you can start to manage your stress. As mentioned earlier, stress produces cortisol, which acidifies your pH level. Often, when people realize that their stress level is affecting their bones, they find it easier to take action to try to control this.

As I discussed earlier, activities like meditation, tai chi, and yoga are very helpful for dealing with stress. Listening to different types of music and brainwave audio recordings are also helpful. There have been many sections in this book that discuss stress-related issues and how to handle stress. It's important to find a way to force negativity from your life that works for you. This will help you with osteoporosis and just about every other aspect of your life.

As for calcium supplements as an effective treatment, the myth about their powers has already been dispelled here, as well as in earlier chapters. It doesn't matter how much calcium you take if you still have that imbalance. If you continue to eat a highly acidic diet and live with too much stress, calcium will not even slightly relieve your bone loss.

For the rare few in our population who are in actual need of calcium, be aware that the body doesn't recognize inorganic materials, which are common in many calcium supplements. As with all supplements, if you are supplementing with calcium, be sure to consume organic calcium and avoid synthetics, and make sure that you consume ionic trace minerals.

Your activity level also plays a key role in the prevention and reversal of bone density loss. Remaining active with weight-bearing exercise is important not only for joint health, as I discussed earlier, but also for bone strength. Some examples of valuable exercises include things like walking and gardening, as well as more rigorous exercise.

Knowledge Is Power

Put down the prescription. You don't need it. The only thing you need to do is educate yourself about what you're doing to acidify your pH level, and then stop doing it.

Always keep the big picture in mind by following the Complete Healing Formula™. Some tweaks to your diet, a little stress relief, and a few less toxins in your environment can mean the difference between brittle bones and brawny bones. Don't sit idly by, assuming you just have to continue to suffer with increasing pain and bone loss. It doesn't have to be that way, and understanding this simple fact is the most important thing of all.

Recommended Resources

Save Our Bones

Get access to more information, research, and tips for bone density loss prevention and treatment from Vivian Goldschmidt's *Save Our Bones* program at http://saveourbones.com.

The Calcium Lie and The Calcium Lie II by Dr. Robert Thompson

Dr. Robert Thompson's books, *The Calcium Lie* and *The Calcium Lie II*, also go into great depth on the subject of bone strength and all the minerals needed for healthy bones. Learn more at www.calciumliebook.com .

CHAPTER 20:

The End of Fibromyalgia

What Is Fibromyalgia?

Fibromyalgia is more than an illness of the body.

When you have fibromyalgia, you suffer from fatigue and pain, but you also experience a tremendous loss of vitality. You can't do the things you want to do and live the life you want to live. Everyone wants a life full of creativity and abundance, but unless we have the energy to make that happen, it's out of reach. Fibromyalgia robs us of that energy.

Because fibromyalgia seems to be on the rise, I have interviewed several experts on this topic. As usual, by understanding the cause of the disease, we can better find solutions. Among the experts whose research and guidance I have found useful are Dr. Greg Fors, Dr. Jacob Teitelbaum, and Dr. Hal Blatman. Much of the information you'll read below comes from these three experts.

Dr. Greg Fors, author of *Why We Hurt: A Complete Physical and Spiritual Guide to Healing Your Chronic Pain,* gave me an excellent analogy to understand fibromyalgia. Imagine the way you feel when you are tired, listless, nauseated, and have a headache. Now imagine living that way every day, all the time. Or imagine that you worked yourself to a place of complete physical and mental exhaustion to the point where you couldn't see or think straight.

That's what fibromyalgia feels like—a total a loss of vitality.

Fibromyalgia is more common than most of us think. It is a widespread pain syndrome affecting approximately ten million diagnosed Americans as of 2014. Fibromyalgia is ten to twenty times more likely to affect women of child-bearing age. However, it can occur in individuals of both sexes in all age groups.

Fibromyalgia is not a simple disease. It's a syndrome that presents complex symptoms. Beyond chronic pain and fatigue, fibromyalgia sufferers also commonly experience headaches, irritable bowel syndrome, numbness, tingling, restlessness, Lake's syndrome, painful menstruation, depression, anxiety, memory cognitive problems, morning stiffness, and many other things. All of these issues drain vitality and keep us from living life to the fullest.

Fibromyalgia may have certain triggers, but it doesn't set in all at once. Many people first start to register it as chronic pain in the back, neck, and shoulders. That pain then snowballs into a widespread pain syndrome until it eventually becomes the serious and debilitating disorder of fibromyalgia. Worse, the same pattern can lead to other degenerative diseases down the line. That's why it's critical to start addressing your fibromyalgia at its root as soon as possible.

What are the myths and lies of fibromyalgia? What are its true causes? And what can you do to resolve the issue from the ground up, using the Complete Healing Formula™ and the concepts of homeostasis, excess, deficiency, and stagnation? This chapter will cover all of these things and more.

The Myths and Lies of Fibromyalgia

One big "lie" regarding fibromyalgia is that it is oftentimes a "trashcan diagnosis."

The term "trashcan diagnosis" has two different meanings, both of which are applicable here. One meaning suggests that there is clearly something wrong, but the doctor can't identify a clear medical problem, and therefore suggests a diagnosis to alleviate the patient's concerns before prescribing something—usually anti-depressants and anti-inflammatories in the case of fibromyalgia.

The second interpretation of the term "trashcan diagnosis" has a more negative connotation. In this line of thought, some believe—incorrectly—that fibromyalgia is a diagnosis given to a set of symptoms stemming from a condition that isn't able to be addressed.

Any way you look at it, however, a "trashcan diagnosis" of fibromyalgia is neither helpful nor accurate. This ailment is real, and it is treatable.

Unfortunately, except for the rare exception of a better-informed doctor, patients with fibromyalgia often receive sub-par help and are left with a feeling of helplessness on top of the already severe symptoms of their illness.

People visit their doctors and say that they're aching and tired. The first things those doctors hand their patients are prescriptions for anti-depressants and anti-inflammatory drugs.

Do these drugs address the problem? No. On the contrary, they make the true causes of fibromyalgia a deeper issue.

Another myth about this illness is that it was once considered a sleep disorder. When you are sore all over, generally you feel more fatigued. However, research now shows that fibromyalgia is not a sleep disorder, and to call it one is a terrible misnomer. Sleep medications have been proven not to be the answer.

In that case, where does the real answer lie?

The True Causes of Fibromyalgia

The real underlying causes of fibromyalgia are nutritional, metabolic, chemical, and emotional. It is important to understand where in the body fibromyalgia pain originates as a result of excesses, deficiencies, and stagnations in these areas.

As I have discussed in earlier chapters, the body is composed of fibroblast cells that form the fascia, connecting and surrounding every muscle fiber and bone in the body. Your fascia in turn forms a communication network throughout your body that integrates your muscles, bones, nervous system, endocrine system, and immune system. Those suffering from fibromyalgia pain are experiencing injury to the fascia, inflammation from food, and a body that is essentially decompensating in many ways.

As we move into the twenty-first century, fibromyalgia is on the rise. I mentioned earlier that at least ten million people were diagnosed with this condition as of 2014, while more than ninety million people with chronic pain and myofascial pain were also estimated to be affected.

According to Dr. Fors, a big part of the reason for the huge numbers and rise in the condition is that our diets have changed drastically in the past several decades. We eat a diet of overconsumption (excess) and under-nutrition (deficiency). In short, we consume more calories than we need, but they are empty calories. This effectively creates a whole population of what Fors calls "the walking wounded."

What's more, our exposure to dangerous chemicals has gone through the roof. The EPA's multi-year studies found traces of some of the deadliest known chemicals in every human being it tested, including dioxin and styrene. Dioxin alone is a chemical used to break down petro chemicals in pesticides and herbicides, and it's estimated that a thimble full of it would kill off New York City. As a neuroendocrine disruptor, dioxin interrupts the functioning of the nervous system and the endocrine system, disrupting the natural flow of our bodies.

These chemicals are ubiquitous. We are eating, drinking, and breathing these very potent toxins. And that does some terrible damage to our tissues and our neuro-immune endocrine systems.

In addition to our terrible diets and exposure to chemicals, Dr. Fors cites two other key causes of fibromyalgia in his research: excess chronic inflammation and oxidative stress.

Why You Feel Pain: Chronic Inflammation and Oxidative Stress

As I explained in previous chapters, inflammation alone is not the problem. Acute inflammation—such as spraining your ankle or getting an infection from a cut—is actually a healing process. Inflammation increases blood flow to the tissue, introducing white blood cells to repair the damage, whether that damage is whiplash, injury, or infection. Without this kind of inflammation, you and I would die.

However, chronic inflammation is a different story. This occurs when the body is unable to turn off its inflammation response. When this happens, it leads to a host of pain and other health issues. Chronic inflammation is what leads to oxidative stress.

Oxidation is like inflammation: we don't want to shut it down completely, because that's how we produce energy. It comes to us through very simple things like exercising and eating healthy foods. However, when taken beyond their natural limits, pro-oxidants in your tissues can damage the body. Oxidative stress may be internal, or it may come from external sources such as pesticides, herbicides, pollution, and other chemicals.

The question you may be asking now is, "Why do I have pain from these things?"

As Dr. Fors explains, the chemicals that your body produces during the inflammatory process stimulate something in your body called "nociceptors," more commonly known as pain receptors. Whenever they feel stress, nociceptors are responsible for firing pain signals up your spinal cord, to your brain, and finally, to your cortex. When those signals reach your cortex, you feel the pain.

Again, nociceptors are a protective response: if you are stressing your tissues, you want to know about it before you damage them. It's when you stress those tissues over and over again that you start to experience problems. The more you activate your nociceptors, the more pain they expect to feel. This causes a physiological change in your spinal cord that makes it more sensitive to detecting pain over time.

Both chronic inflammation and oxidative stress are metabolic issues, and they are strongly interconnected. You can't have one without the other. They are two of the major underpinnings of chronic pain disorders like fibromyalgia. And eventually, they lead to the true cause of the loss of vitality that fibromyalgia sufferers experience: mitochondrial decline.

Mitochondria: Power Plants of the Cell

Mitochondria are fascinating little organelles. They are the power plants of our cells, and each cell needs thousands of mitochondria to function optimally.

Mitochondria produce something called ATP, which Dr. Fors refers to as the "energy currency" we use on a daily basis, whether we are hugging our families, thinking a thought, or eating lunch. Whatever we do, we have to buy that action with ATP. Each of us produces our body weight in ATP each day, and we use it up immediately.

Now imagine if your mitochondria aren't producing as much ATP as they should. Nutrient-deficient diets, exposure to chemicals, and simple genetics can all prevent our mitochondria for getting what they need to produce ATP. Without ATP, we have no energy currency. And without energy, we lose our vitality. This is the scenario that takes place in the case of fibromyalgia.

Trigger Mechanism

Another true cause of fibromyalgia is that it is often kicked off by some kind of trigger mechanism.

In one piece of literature on the subject, 42 percent of women with fibromyalgia had first suffered a whiplash injury. That injury was not corrected properly up front, and the result was excess chronic inflammation and oxidative stress. Moreover, their tissues were stressed to begin with because they had been eating nutrient-deficient diets. They had inadvertently set themselves up for metabolic dysfunction, and so the stage was set for chronic pain.

You may not even be aware of your trigger mechanism, because it wasn't something that you realized would result in a lifetime of pain. Even powerful emotions—such as those caused by the death of a spouse—can play a major role in triggering fibromyalgia.

Dysbiosis

Still another cause of fibromyalgia is dysbiosis, an imbalance of microbes in the body.

In his research on the disease, Mark Pimentel measured a group of fibromyalgia patients for the amount of bad bacteria growing in their guts. He discovered that 100 percent of fibromyalgia patients contained these bad microbes.

Dysbiosis is one of the largest reservoirs for pro-oxidants and chronic inflammation, and those who suffer from it should take probiotics, magnesium, and other supplements to rectify the issue.

Negative Emotions

Finally, as with all other physical ailments, there is a strong connection between emotions and chronic pain like fibromyalgia.

As I discussed earlier, emotions affect the area of your brain called the amygdala that regulates things like fear, anger, rage, and pain. This is the center of your emotional brain, or limbic system. When your amygdala communicates with the conscious part of your brain—the pre-frontal cortex—and the message between them is "Oh my gosh, this is terrible," the part of your brain that helps to govern pain is activated.

This can become a vicious cycle. Negative thoughts and emotions release peptides that cause us to become addicted to our own negativity. As a result, we continue with the same negative patterns, just because we are comfortable with the way we are feeling.

Nutrition-deficient diets, exposure to chemicals, mitochondrial degeneration, trigger mechanisms, dysbiosis, and negative emotions all come together to form the true causes of fibromyalgia. With that in mind, how do we go about treating this degenerative illness?

Effective Treatments for Fibromyalgia

Now you understand that fibromyalgia is a huge syndrome that needs to be addressed in a systematic way on many different fronts. You need to take a holistic, comprehensive approach to this problem. There are many different ways to climb the mountain to recovery, and all of these will help you experience a significant reduction in pain and an improvement in your feeling of vitality.

What can you do to start feeling better today?

Clean Up Your Diet

In his book, *Why We Hurt: A Complete Physical Instruction Guide to Healing Your Chronic Pain*, Dr. Fors advocates a five-step cleanup program. He suggests beginning with a change in diet, passing on unhealthy foods in favor of vegetables and whole grains. Err on the side of a Mediterranean diet. Move toward organic foods as much as possible to reduce your intake of pesticides and herbicides. Filter your water and clean up your personal environment to further minimize your intake of chemicals.

Change Your Body's Oil

Dr. Fors's book also suggests doing an "oil change" to get rid of the hydrogenated oils, saturated fats, many animal fats, and trans fatty acids that promote chronic inflammation. Increase your intake of fish oils, which contain anti-inflammatory omega 3s. This will tune up your cellular engine: your mitochondria. Magnesium, vitamin B complex, thiamine/ginger root and cumin extracts, and turmeric are also great support for the mitochondria.

Get Regular

Maintaining excellent excretory function is another important part of a cleanup program. Two bowel movements a day are ideal in order to remove the toxins from your body. Without proper excretion, toxins back up in your system, which makes fibromyalgia worse. Overcome any issues with dysbiosis by replacing the bad microbes with probiotics.

Eliminate Trigger Points

Dr. Hal Blatman, author of *The Art of Body Maintenance: Winners' Guide to Pain Relief*, emphasizes the treatment of trigger points as a critical part of resolving fibromyalgia and chronic pain. As I discussed in chapter 8, trigger points are knots in your muscle tissue. Trigger points can even alter your nervous system itself along with your muscle tissue. It is critical to address trigger points in addition to metabolic dysfunctions, or you will not get far with resolving your fibromyalgia symptoms.

Trigger points need to be physically removed. Because fibromyalgia sufferers are so sensitive to pain, they need to take this slow and easy. However, working through it yourself is better than having someone treat your pain for you. Seeking treatment from medical professionals is costly and time-consuming: doctors and chiropractors need to be reimbursed for their care, and most insurance companies do not reimburse you for treatment.

By contrast, you can change the underlying physiology of your muscle tissue yourself simply by applying mechanical pressure to the tissue over time. When you apply pressure to a trigger point for up to one minute, the tissue softens, allowing better oxygen and nutrients to flow through it. This washes out toxins and allows your mitochondria to function better, relieving the tight muscle.

Experts agree that anyone can use passive pressure rather than active pressure to treat their trigger points, since the latter puts more strain on the muscles you are trying to relax. You can do this by simply lying down on a hard, raised object, such as a small tennis ball, or by using one of the devices mentioned in chapter 8. When using this type of device, be sure to relax as much as possible by making yourself comfortable: find a pillow or a cushion, put on your favorite TV show, and let the trigger points treat themselves.

If you have fibromyalgia throughout your whole body, treat the upper body one night and the lower body the next. Perform the treatment for around fifteen minutes at a time. It takes about one minute to treat each trigger point, so you can cover a lot of trigger points in a fifteen-minute period. Start with light pressure and move slowly. This form of treatment is not difficult, but it does require discipline to do it with consistency.

By catching trigger points early, you may be able to prevent the spread of pain to the different quadrants of your body. Pay particular attention to this if you have experienced a trigger event like whiplash. Cases of fibromyalgia can arise in as little as six months to a year after such an event.

Change Your Inner Dialogue

Finally, as I have shown from the testimony of many experts on pain earlier in this book, treating the emotional aspect of fibromyalgia by engaging in positive self-talk is critical. If your amygdala is overstimulated from negative emotions, you have the power to change that pattern. Begin to talk to yourself in soothing ways. We can promote a more peaceful state of mind simply by paying attention to how our inner dialogue is going.

Inner dialogue is a powerful self-care therapy device. Tell yourself that you can make a difference to your health, and open yourself up to healing emotions such as forgiveness and gratitude. If you are an individual who is holding on to an injustice or wound from an earlier time in your life, find a way to let it go. Dr. Fors shared a quote with me that I must repeat to you: "forgiveness is giving up all hope of a better past to build a bridge to a better future."

When it comes to treating fibromyalgia, you have to be complete, you have to give it time, and you have to stay disciplined. You can't just throw a little bit of effort at it and expect to come out the other side completely cured. Fibromyalgia treatment requires commitment. When you really commit, you put yourself once more on the path to health.

Fibro Fix

Fibromyalgia may feel like a curse. But it can also be a great blessing if we take the opportunity to learn more about ourselves and how we work. Ask yourself: How did I get here? Look at the excesses, deficiencies, and stagnations in the

Wellness Model of Health™ and say, "What can I do to turn this around?" You may find more vitality and a more fulfilling life than the one you used to live, filled with health and a new appreciation for your abilities.

Recovery from fibromyalgia begins with personal responsibility. Self-care is our best hope. We need to take responsibility for healing ourselves from pain, and our earth from chemicals.

Don't try to relieve the symptoms of your fibromyalgia alone. Heal your pain now, from the source, to prevent more symptoms and other diseases later down the line. Develop the "warrior spirit," love yourself, and overcome this challenge from the inside out. I have seen people achieve this hundreds and thousands of times. You have the power to be next.

Recommended Resources

Why We Hurt: A Complete Physical and Spiritual Guide to Healing Your Chronic Pain by Dr. Greg Fors. Learn more at www.whywehurt.com.

Trigger Point Self-Treatment System
For more information, visit http://www.losethebackpain.com/ triggerpointselftreatment.html.

The Art of Body Maintenance: Winners' Guide to Pain Relief
by Dr. Hal Blatman, MD, and Brad Ekvall, BFA

The Fatigue and Fibromyalgia Solution
Learn more at http://www.endfatigue.com.

CHAPTER 21:

The End of Heart Disease

What Is Heart Disease?

Every year in the United States, about six hundred thousand people die of heart disease. That means that heart disease is the leading cause of death in this country, responsible for 25 percent of its total deaths. Our health care system spends over $108 billion a year on heart disease-related costs, yet the problem is still enormous.

The Mayo Clinic broadly defines heart disease as a wide range of diseases that affect the heart, including blood vessel disease, coronary artery disease, and heart rhythm problems. It is often used synonymously with "cardiovascular disease," which refers only to narrowing or blockage of blood vessels. But however you define it, the end result takes you to the same destination: one where serious complications—and possibly, death—result from the failure of the circulatory system.

As with other conditions, American medicine is built around treating the symptoms of heart disease rather than targeting its underlying causes. I've said it before, and I'll say it again here: it may be called the health care system, but it is really the "sick-care system." While it may be gratifying to know that the United States has the top technology for state-of-the-art treatments, there is almost no economic benefit built anywhere in our system to prevent heart disease. That's where practicing self-health comes into play.

In this chapter, I'll take you through the myths, lies, and truths about heart disease, and show you how you can resolve this disease using the Wellness Model of Health™.

The Myths and Lies of Heart Disease

There is a lot of confusion and misinformation out there when it comes to heart disease. According to Dr. Dwight Lundell, a heart health pioneer who has performed over five thousand heart surgeries and the author of *The*

Cholesterol Lie, much of the generally accepted paradigm for heart disease over the past few decades was scientifically incorrect.

When Dr. Lundell began his career as a heart surgeon in the 1970s, the accepted cause of heart disease was an excess amount of cholesterol in the blood that slowly built up inside the arteries, much like corrosion builds up in the plumbing lines of your house. The solution to the problem was mechanical: detour around the blockages. That was how heart operations came to be known as "bypass surgery."

For some time, surgeons performed angioplasties in which they inserted the equivalent of a little balloon into the artery to squeeze plaque material out of the way. However, after angioplasties began to fail and the artery began to narrow again, the medical community was forced to take a second look at what was really going on. They next inserted a piece of metal into the artery called a stent, which was designed to reduce the failure rate of the angioplasties.

Nevertheless, ten years later, the same people who had heart surgery would be back on the operating table for additional work. One famous example is former president Bill Clinton, who had quadruple coronary bypass surgery in 2004. Shortly after this, he had to have another surgery to fix a complication. And less than six years after that, he was once again back in the hospital to address and resolve more heart issues.

Clinton's life was extended and his symptoms were reduced as a result of the surgeries he underwent, but with him—as with many other heart-disease sufferers—the illness was not cured. Now a well-known vegan, Clinton appears to have had enough surgery and decided to address his health through diet and lifestyle changes—another example of improving health and wellness through restoring homeostasis to the mind, body, and diet.

Perhaps the biggest myth about heart disease is its supposed connection to high cholesterol. Lundell and others have discovered this connection to be inaccurate. In fact, in a study of 137,000 people admitted to US hospitals for heart-related problems in 2008, 75 percent of them demonstrated normal levels of bad LDL cholesterol.

Another big lie about heart disease is its relationship to saturated and animal fats. For many years, these fats were assumed to contribute to heart disease based on the fact that they might raise cholesterol. However, in Dr. Lundell's research, he reviewed several big population studies on the subject and discovered that there wasn't a single shred of evidence connecting saturated fat to heart disease.

In fact, ironically, if you don't get enough saturated fats, you can end up having a stroke. Recall the Rosetans in Pennsylvania. Their heart problems were non-existent when they were eating animal fats, and only began to climb when they changed their diets to follow the myths of the accepted "heart-healthy" diet.

With the accepted medical paradigm of heart disease falling apart in the face of new science, what are the true causes of this illness?

The True Causes of Heart Disease

The truth about cholesterol and what it takes to have a healthy heart may surprise you.

According to Dr. Lundell, as a result of failing angioplasties and coronary bypasses, people began to take a second look at what was really going on inside our arteries. They discovered that, rather than particles of cholesterol collecting in our arteries, that cholesterol—along with other matter like calcium and scar tissue—were actually within the wall of the blood vessel, comprising what we call "plaque." Furthermore, the place where cholesterol collected first was inside our white blood cells.

The question then arose, why would cholesterol be inside of white blood cells? Researchers realized that cholesterol was in those white blood cells because of inflammation. Anti-inflammatory chemicals called cytokines were activating them. Without inflammation, the white blood cells would never accumulate cholesterol, and it would never gather in the walls of our blood vessels at all.

From this we can see that the quantity of cholesterol is not really the issue, as we previously thought. Cholesterol only becomes a problem when it is either oxidized or has a sugar molecule attached to it. Under those circumstances, our white blood cells perceive the cholesterol as abnormal and try to consume it. However, they can't dissolve the cholesterol after they've absorbed it. This is the real root cause of plaque.

We can also see how chronic inflammation is such an important factor when understanding the true source of heart disease. Inside of our blood vessels is a very thin, delicate single-cell layer of tissue called the endothelium. If we were to spread this endothelium out, it would cover between eight and ten tennis courts of surface area.

Blood circulates through our systems very rapidly: our whole blood volume travels through our bodies three or four times per minute, depending on our activity level. Because of this, any chemical that's consumed by one part of our body rapidly spreads to the other areas. In other words, if we have a chronic injury somewhere in a blood vessel, the inflammatory response quickly becomes widespread, and this marks the beginnings of plaque buildup.

We do physical damage to our blood vessels in any number of ways. Smoking is one example. The chemicals we inhale from smoking quickly circulate through the rest of our bodies, causing chronic injury to the blood vessels. This is why people who smoke cigarettes end up with lots of plaque disease in their arteries, in addition to lung cancer. The smoke causes a chronic inflammatory response.

What we need to do, then, is look at what causes excessive injury to our blood vessels on a repeated and regular basis. What makes our cholesterol appear abnormal to our white blood cells, causing those cells to consume them and resulting in chronic inflammation and plaque buildup? What in our environments is causing this injury on a consistent basis?

When I interviewed Dr. Lundell for my *Live Pain Free* newsletter, he shared with me the four primary sources of chronic inflammation that adversely affect our heart health: sugar, soybean oil, a lack of Omega-3 fatty acids, and oxidative stress.

Sugars

A century ago, the average American consumed very little sugar. Less than one hundred years later, we now consume seventeen times the amount of sugar that people did back then. In America, the average consumption of sugar has skyrocketed to 170 pounds a year—almost half a pound a day. We simply don't think about it, but sugar is a major excess in our diets.

Consider this: one can of soda contains nine teaspoons of sugar. No parent would allow his or her child to sit down with a sugar bowl and eat nine teaspoons of sugar. Yet most of us have all bought our children and grandchildren Cokes or Pepsis at some time or another without a second thought.

Our sugar consumption extends to our carbohydrates. Most Americans consume a high-carbohydrate diet, because since the 1970s we have been encouraged to reduce fat in our diets and replace them with carbs. Pastas, breakfast cereals, and other carbohydrates all contribute to our consumption of sugar.

What happens in our bodies when we consume excessive sugar? Picture the keyboard on your computer. Now imagine that you dump syrup over it. This causes it to become sticky and difficult to use. The same thing happens inside us when we inundate our bodies with sugar: we get sticky, and things don't work as well as they should. Our excess calories create oxidative stress that damages our proteins and needs to be cleaned up.

There is no question that our high intake of carbohydrates is a leading cause of heart disease and premature death.

Soybean Oil

The next major culprit of chronic inflammation on Dr. Lundell's list is the excess consumption of soybean oil.

Soybean oil was never part of the human diet until the middle of the twentieth century. When people first began to grow concerned about heart disease, they were intimidated by the idea that animal fat raised cholesterol, and that cholesterol was responsible for the illness. The Department of Agriculture and the original Food Pyramid therefore recommended avoiding all animal fats and suggest replacing those animal fats with plant oils.

This gave rise to soybean and corn oils, which now permeate grocery store shelves and are found in a multitude of pre-packaged and processed foods.

Originally, they were intended to make us healthier. However, we later discovered that these oils contain large amounts of Omega-6 free fatty acids.

Omega-6 fatty acids are metabolized into pro-inflammatory cytokines. The result is that they start pouring chemicals into our circulation that get our bodies more geared up for an inflammatory result than they should be. This in turn activates excessive white blood cells, which begin consuming the bad LDL cholesterol and forming plaque.

I'll borrow a great analogy from my interview with Dr. Lundell to explain this: consuming soybean oil is like throwing sand into part of your motor. No matter how fast you rev the motor, the inflammation is going to continue destroying your regular tissues, and they will never have a chance to heal.

Fried things, baked goods, and many other things with long shelf lives often contain soybean oils. In fact, as of 2014, it was estimated that teenagers could be getting as many as 20 percent of their daily calories from soybean oil simply because of their consumption of french fries.

To make matters worse, taxpayers subsidize the production of soybeans, which makes soybean oil cheap and easy to purchase. It is everywhere, and it is in everything, making it difficult to avoid. This is one of the big reasons why soybean oil is such an insidious invader of our health.

Lack of Omega-3s

The third major cause of inflammation affecting heart disease is a deficiency of Omega-3 essential free fatty acids in our bodies. The term "essential" means that we don't produce these fatty acids naturally; we need to get them from our diets. The Omega-6 free fatty acids that I discussed in the last section are not essential; our bodies already produce them, which is why we need to consume a small amount of Omega-6 to supplement that natural production.

Historically, many years ago, our consumption of Omega-3 to Omega-6 fatty acids had a ratio of about one to one. As of 2014, that dietary ratio had become almost one to twenty, Omega-6 over Omega-3. The reason this is important is that Omega-3 fatty acids are metabolized into anti-inflammatory chemicals in our bodies. Once metabolized, they compete with enzymes against pro-inflammatory Omega-6 fatty acids. Without adequate Omega-3 intake to balance the influence of Omega-6, the stage is set for inflammation.

About 80 percent of the US population is deficient in Omega-3s. While we get a few more Omega-3s from grass-fed, free-range animals and animal products like milk and eggs, these still aren't enough. This is why getting enough high-quality fish oil, either from a good supplement or from eating fish, is such an important factor when it comes to reducing inflammation in the body.

Omega-3 essential fatty acids affect more than just heart health. They also affect our brains. These oils are fats, and the human brain is composed of about 60 percent fat. Omega-3s make up the cell membranes of our brain cells, which means that making sure we get enough of this important fatty acid can only help our state of health.

What's more, Omega-3s have proven behavioral implications. For example, in one prison population in England, the addition of an Omega-3 supplement to the inmates reduced violence by 60 percent. In schools, children who consume more Omega-3s in their diets experience fewer behavior and attention-deficit problems.

The powerful influence of Omega-3s extends to many ailments. Dr. Lundell shared a study with me showing that patients with rheumatoid arthritis were able to cut their medication doses in half simply by consuming reasonable doses of fish oil supplements.

Post-partum depression was reduced to almost zero when mothers supplemented their pregnancies with fish oils, and the children of these mothers showed higher intelligence levels and motor skills than children whose mothers did not take fish oil. Other kinds of depression can also be alleviated by adding the proper amount of Omega-3s to our diets.

With a list of benefits like this, we can see why the lack of Omega-3 essential fatty acids in our bodies would result in poor heart health, among other problems.

Oxidative Stress

The fourth major cause of inflammation that affects heart disease is an excess of oxidative stress.

I talked a little bit about oxidative stress and its relationship to chronic inflammation in the last chapter. We are creatures that need oxygen to live, and as a consequence of this, we produce free radicals. Free radicals are molecules that have lost an electron. That molecule then becomes unstable and goes out to steal an electron from its neighbor. When too many of these unstable molecules come together in our tissues, we develop oxidative stress.

Oxidative stress is strongly connected to injury and inflammation. The more chronic injury and inflammation we have, the more free radicals and oxidative stress we produce, and this is a major cause of chronic illness such as heart disease.

This is why we need to get more antioxidants in our diets. To balance our production of free radicals, our bodies also produce antioxidants to combat them. However, we need to get the building blocks to produce antioxidants in the first place, or we can't keep up that balance. We get the building blocks for antioxidants from an amino acid called cysteine, which we find in foods like milk and meat. Populations that eat a lot of vegetables also have less overall oxidative stress.

What causes excess oxidative stress? According to Dr. Lundell, a number of things contribute to this problem. Excess calorie intake is a big culprit, particularly when we consume too much sugar. Irritations like cigarette smoking are also big contributors. Chemicals in the body that we take in from our environment and insufficient exercise are also factors. But the biggest source of oxidative stress is dietary deficiency—not getting the building blocks we need to produce the antioxidants we need to combat this kind of stress.

Emotional Components

The body and diet alone aren't the only things that lead to heart disease. As we saw in tight-knit communities like that of the Rosetans, where family and community support are strong, lower levels of stress directly correlate with low levels of heart disease and coronary infarctions. We're back to the third component of the Complete Healing Formula™: the mind. And it makes a lot of sense.

As we feel more stress, especially chronic stress, our blood vessels tighten and our breathing becomes rapid and shallow. You've already seen the impact of this in earlier chapters. The bottom line is that the same emotional stress that constricts our blood vessels, when left unchecked for a long time, will inevitably lead to a greater incidence of heart-related diseases.

Forging strong bonds of support with family and the community will go a long way toward improved heart health. In addition, developing healthy emotional habits to deal with stress and planning for regular relaxation will further aid you in your quest for better heart health.

Effective Treatment and Prevention for Heart Disease

There comes a time when heart disease progresses to the point that emergency measures must be taken. Even Dr. Lundell admits that heart surgeries are sometimes necessary; he is, after all, a heart surgeon. However, remember that unless you are in the middle of a heart attack, you can take action to begin to reverse the damage inflicted on your heart right away.

It's important to note that many things classified as heart disease are really risk factors or causes of major, catastrophic health events. By making preventative changes and adjusting your diet, lifestyle, and emotional habits, damage to your heart can be stopped and reversed many times over.

We can work to prevent heart disease by following Dr. Lundell's recommendations for avoiding chronic inflammation. Consume less sugar in your diet. Avoid products made with soybean oils. Increase your intake of Omega-3 essential fatty acids, whether from high-quality supplements or from consuming more healthy fish. Reduce your levels of oxidative stress by upping your antioxidants. Increase your intake of vitamin C. And don't forget to relax.

So often, it takes a very long time to uncover the true underlying causes of an illness and to address those true causes, rather than just managing symptoms. Heart disease is no exception. When you follow the guidelines outlined above, you can finally begin to heal your heart disease in a real and lasting sense, using the Wellness Model of Health™.

Recommended Resources

The Great Cholesterol Lie by Dwight Lundell
Learn more at www.thecholesterollie.com.

The Power of Clan: The Influence of Human Relationships on Heart Disease by Stewart Wolf and John G. Bruhn

The Calcium Lie II by Dr. Robert Thompson
Learn more at www.calciumliebook.com

CHAPTER 22:

The End of Cancer

What Is Cancer?

Cancer is the second largest cause of death in the United States. The American Cancer Society estimated that over 1.6 million new cancer cases would be diagnosed and over 580,000 people would die of this disease in 2014. According to the National Institute of Health, as a nation, we spent an estimated $216.6 billion on this disease alone in 2009.

The American Cancer Society defines cancer as "a group of diseases characterized by the uncontrolled growth and spread of abnormal cells." What is less well-known among the general public is that organs and tissues in the body produce these abnormal cells all the time, and the body usually suppresses, quarantines, or kills them. In the case of cancer, however, something prevents the body's natural defense mechanisms from eliminating these abnormal cells.

Why, then, doesn't the general medical community seek out natural alternatives to toxic treatments like chemotherapy? Unfortunately, it's not due to a lack of success with natural treatments. The groups earning billions of dollars to research chemical and radioactive agents don't want to lose that money. The same health care economy that pushes drugs that merely treat symptoms keeps this failed model moving forward.

As I said before, health care in the United States has become a business of astounding proportions. Big pharmaceutical companies have an enormous financial interest in preserving current cancer treatments, despite the fact that those treatments entail chemicals and radiation that are themselves proven carcinogens. They're so focused on protecting their turf economically that they turn a blind eye—and even actively fight against—other opportunities and options that are emerging for the treatment of cancer.

This chapter will take you through the current myths and lies about cancer. It will also give you fascinating information regarding the true underlying causes of this disease, along with actions you can take to start fighting cancer using the Wellness Model of Health™ today.

The Myths and Lies of Cancer

Even though we know the statistics, there is a lot of misinformation out there about the true causes of cancer.

The first myth relates to what many people believe to be the cause or start of cancer. This myth states that normal cells become cancer cells when there is damage to the DNA in the cell. Unlike other cells that die, these damaged cells remain alive and reproduce. Over time, the damaged or genetically mutated cells form a tumor, which then spreads throughout the body via the bloodstream.

However, the truth is that there is no explanation of how a cell's DNA becomes mutated in the first place, except in cases where there is a genetic mutation already present. Building on the work of Dr. John Beard and Dr. William Donald Kelley, Dr. Nicholas J. Gonzalez offers an amazing discovery that is not widely publicized by the medical community. According to Dr. Gonzalez, rather than forming from a mutation in the cells of the tissue (or mature cells), cancer begins from primitive, undifferentiated cells—what we now know as "stem cells."

Another common misconception about cancer is rooted in truth, but then strays from an effective treatment of the causes. Modern science gives us a long list of cancer causes, including infectious organisms, tobacco, hormones, immune conditions, chemicals, radiation, and both inherited and metabolic mutations. This list of causes is actually quite accurate. As I discussed in earlier chapters, the presence of toxins can indeed lead to diseases, and tobacco, chemicals, and radiation surely fit the bill as toxins. I also reviewed the impact of parasites on ill-health.

The "myth" element comes into play when we look at the medical community's proposed "solutions" to the cancer caused by these toxins.

Common treatments for cancer involve surgically removing the tumor, or blasting the tumor (and all surrounding healthy tissues) with toxins such as chemicals and radiation. If cancer cells were "good guys gone bad," blasting them to dust would solve the problem, albeit with some collateral damage. However, this treatment fails to account for the fact that the cancer doesn't develop from the tissue's differentiated cells, but rather from natural, omnipresent stem cells.

Therefore, the accepted treatments simply eliminate the symptoms of cancer—the tumors—without addressing its cause: why the stem cells weren't kept in check to begin with, as is normally the case. Many people have had firsthand experience of a loved one whose cancer went into remission, only to suddenly return at a later date.

Thankfully, pioneering doctors have identified more than just the toxins and parasites involved in cancer development. They have also discovered the mechanisms we can use to keep the growth of cancer in check.

The True Causes of Cancer

Most experts agree that we all produce cancer cells every day, and these cells can be the origin of cancer as we know it. In recent years, three pioneering researchers have made groundbreaking discoveries that have shed new light on the true causes of cancer. Dr. Nicholas J. Gonzalez, Dr. Stanislaw Burzynski, and Dr. Hulda Clark each bring to the table a unique understanding of the causes and—ultimately—the cures for cancer.

Through both his own research and reviewing the work of Dr. John Beard from the early 1900s, Dr. Gonzalez realized that the cells that eventually form cancer aren't what the medical community has believed them to be. As mentioned above, Gonzalez asserts that cancers do not develop from mutations in normal tissue cells. Rather, they develop from the lack of control of primitive, undifferentiated stem cells.

These stem cells, which have been all the rage in medical headlines in recent years, exist and work throughout the body all the time. For example, your skin heals after a cut because the body activates—or more accurately, sets free—stem cells to rebuild the damaged tissue and skin. The scab, essentially an overgrowth, is then cleaned away by the body, leaving hopefully unscarred new skin behind.

It is this fact that really sets the stage for understanding the true causes of cancer. Something has to set the stem cells free, and something has to stop them from acting normally when the time comes. It is along this line of thinking that the groundbreaking work of Dr. Burzynski and Dr. Clark sheds some light.

In the 1970s, after obtaining his PhD from Lublin Medical University at the age of twenty-four, Dr. Stanislaw Burzynski made a fascinating observation: individuals with cancer were deficient in a certain strain of peptides in their blood and urine that healthy people had in abundance.

Dr. Burzynski found a way to extract the missing peptides from healthy donors and began treating terminally ill cancer patients with these. In this way, he began working toward restoring homeostasis in the cancer patients' body systems. He called his method "gene-targeted therapy," because his approach targeted cancer-causing genes in the human body using antineoplastons.

Gene-targeted therapy works by "switching on" a higher level of genes in the body that work to suppress cancer cells. Essentially, he found a mechanism that activated and deactivated the stem cells, keeping them dormant when they were not needed.

Dr. Burzynski's innovative approach was entirely new way to treat cancer, and the results were impressive. In 2005, a clinical trial using traditional radiation and chemotherapy techniques reported that only five out of fifty-four participants ended up cancer-free—a success rate of 9 percent. By contrast, a 2008 trial using Burzynski's antineoplastons reported that five out of twenty-five participants emerged cancer-free from the treatment—a success rate of 25 percent.

In other words, standard cancer treatment protocol was over 60 percent less successful than Burzynski's treatment. What's more, the second group of participants experienced no negative side effects from their treatment. It's no surprise that the medical community, funded by expensive radiation and chemotherapy drugs, didn't latch onto a treatment that uses something that occurs naturally, and therefore can't be sold for a big profit.

Another major breakthrough into the true underlying causes of cancer was discovered by Dr. Hulda Clark, whose research I discussed in detail in earlier chapters. In her book, *The Cure for All Cancers,* Dr. Clark asserts that cancer is actually caused by parasites —in particular, flatworms. Flatworms commonly live in the intestines of humans and other species. Clark states that when these flatworms lay eggs that are not passed out of the body through bowel movements, the groundwork for cancer is laid.

Cancer itself then appears when these eggs are exposed to propyl alcohol, a common ingredient in many of our household items, including shampoos, cosmetics, mouthwash, rubbing alcohol, shaving supplies, white sugar, and even bottled water. The slightest exposure to propyl alcohol in any form acts as a catalyst for flatworm eggs to develop, and a few batches of larvae multiply into hundreds more within a short period of time.

According to Dr. Clark, different types of cancer are simply a question of location. If the parasite eggs develop in the breast, the result is breast cancer. If they develop in the prostate, this becomes prostate cancer, and so forth.

Carcinogens, which are commonly thought to cause cancer, actually act like magnets for cancer, drawing the parasites to different areas of the body. In her book, Clark gives the example that nickel causes prostate cancer by attracting parasites to that organ of the body. In addition to nickel, she also strongly cautions against exposure to Freon, copper, fiberglass or asbestos, mercury, lead, and formaldehyde.

Clark's approach agrees that some toxins and carcinogens facilitate cancer, and she asserts that they do so by drawing the offending parasites to a particular area in the body, setting off a chain of events that allows the cancer to spread.

In light of the true causes of this widespread disease, what can we do to effectively treat and prevent cancer?

Effective Treatment and Prevention for Cancer

While specialized treatment methods such as those performed by Dr. Stanislaw Burzynski can be effective, they are also time consuming and expensive, and they require a specialist who is willing to perform the procedure, which can be difficult if not impossible to find.

Dr. Gonzalez and Dr. Clark, however, offer several effective points of advice that you can follow in order to play an active role in your own cancer treatment and prevention.

Gonzalez Protocol

Dr. Gonzalez's therapy basically involves three components: diet, aggressive supplementation with nutrients and pancreas product (containing naturally occurring enzymes), and detoxification.

These protocols are individualized on a case-by-case basis. Following Dr. Gonzalez's analysis, each patient receives a diet plan that is designed for his or her specific needs. The diets are quite variable, ranging from a pure vegetarian program to a diet requiring fatty red meat two to three times a day.

Gonzalez's intense supplement regimens are also individualized: each cancer patient consumes between 130 and 175 capsules daily. Non-cancer patients require considerably fewer supplements per day. The supplement regimens include a range of vitamins, minerals, trace elements, anti-oxidants, and animal glandular products, prescribed according to the particular patient's needs and cancer type.

The nutrients from the supplement regimens are not believed to have a direct anti-cancer effect. Rather, they serve to improve overall metabolic function to help the body fight the good fight. This aligns perfectly with the concept of achieving homeostasis between mind, body, and diet. In addition to these supplements, every cancer patient takes large quantities of pancreas product in capsule form, which is believed to contribute the main anti-cancer action.

The third component of Dr. Gonzalez's protocol involves detoxification routines. Dr. Gonzalez found that as patients repaired and rebuilt their systems, large amounts of metabolic waste and stored toxins were released. As a result, patients routinely developed a variety of symptoms, most commonly described as "flu-like," such as low grade fevers, muscle aches and pains, and even rashes. Detoxification works to ease and prevent these negative effects from stored toxins.

You can learn more about Dr. Gonzalez's methods in the Recommended Resources section at the end of this chapter.

Clark Protocol

Dr. Clark points out that the appearance of cancer is a recipe with two ingredients: intestinal fluke parasites and propyl alcohol. Without both of these components, cancer cannot develop.

Therefore, even if you have parasites like flatworms in your system, the onset of cancer will not commence as long as you avoid exposure to propyl alcohol. Once you stop your intake of propyl alcohol, Clark says that all traces of the substance will be gone from your body in three days or less.

In addition to avoiding propyl alcohol, Dr. Clark recommends ridding yourself of the parasites themselves using herbal treatments and the "zapping" method, as covered earlier. Clark asserts that you can stop cancer malignancy by using a frequency generator on your body for three-minute intervals at several different frequencies, which are listed in her book. Once the parasite growth factors have been eliminated in this manner, she says, they will not return unless you reintroduce new parasites into your system.

Even after you eliminate the root of the cancer, Dr. Clark points out that you may still have to address any effects that it had on the rest of your body while it was active in order to fully return your system to its natural state of homeostasis. Dr. Clark recommends removing toxins from the affected organs and then allowing the body to take its natural course in repairing the damage done by the cancer.

Because cancer is caused by parasites, Dr. Clark cautions that you need to stay vigilant against picking up parasites from a wide range of sources. Undercooked meats and dairy products, pets, and even other people—including family members—all make an appearance on Dr. Clark's list of potential carriers. According to Dr. Clark, you can reinfect yourself with parasites even through something as seemingly simple and innocent as a kiss.

Avoid infecting yourself with new fluke parasites by making sure that all of your meat and dairy products are thoroughly cooked. You can remove parasites from your pets using the natural pet parasite program outlined in Clark's book. Also work to eliminate toxins from your environment to your maximum ability.

Dr. Clark cautions that if you are suffering from cancer, the rest of your family is very likely carrying the same fluke parasites in their intestines. Those recovering from cancer should ask their family members to undergo the same herbal and zapping treatments they perform on themselves in order to reduce the risk of reinfection.

Finally, Dr. Clark strongly encourages a high consumption of vitamin C in the treatment and prevention of cancer. Refer back to chapters 11 and 15 to read more about toxins and cleanses. Although propyl alcohol is the catalyst for cancer, our bodies are designed to detoxify it. Those who develop cancer bypass this natural detoxification system because of the presence of aflatoxin—a mold that is found in common foods such as fruit and bread.

Vitamin C destroys aflatoxin, and because of that it can be a powerful tool in the prevention of cancer. Dr. Clark recommends taking 500 mg of vitamin C with each meal. Other experts, including Dr. Thompson, encourage even higher doses of vitamin C in your diet.

The combination of parasites, toxins, and aflatoxin building up in our systems over the years is the platform from which cancer takes flight.

It's no coincidence that all three of these experts—Drs. Gonzalez, Burzynski, and Clark—approach cancer from the angle of restoring homeostasis to the body. This just goes to show that the Wellness Model of Health™ is the solution that lies beneath even the most serious diseases we face as a nation. When we work to remove the causes of cancer, we can treat and prevent this terrible condition at its source.

Recommended Resources

The Cure for All Diseases by Dr. Hulda Clark

Cancer Is a Dangerous Business, a documentary by Dr. Stanislaw Burzynski

Enzymes and Cancer (DVD):
For more information, visit http://www.amazon.com/Enzymes-Cancer-Nicholas-J-Gonzalez/dp/B001OI36GW.

What Went Wrong: The Truth behind the Clinical Trial of the Enzyme Treatment of Cancer by Dr. Nicholas Gonzalez

Beating Cancer with Nutrition by Patrick Quillin

PART III:

The Future of Healthy, Pain-Free Living

CHAPTER 23:

Your Roadmap to Optimal Health and Wellness

The Truth about Wellness

Now you know the truth about wellness. By understanding the real causes of pain and illness, and by taking action to rectify them using the Wellness Model of Health™ and the Complete Healing Formula™, you can overcome even the gravest health conditions. You can eliminate pain, prevent and cure diseases, reinstate happiness, and embrace each day with optimism and satisfaction.

You can reclaim a healthy, vibrant life.

The health plagues on our society are real—but so are their cures. No one has more stake in your health than you. When you take responsibility for and control of your own wellness outcomes, you empower yourself to find the healing answers you have been searching for.

The journey back to health is rewarding, though in some cases it may also be a long and challenging road. You don't have to travel that road alone. The Healthy Back Institute and *Live Pain Free* are committed to giving you the information and tools you need to relieve your pain, cure your disease, and rediscover a life of fullness and enrichment.

In this chapter, I have gathered together a wealth of resources to jumpstart your journey to wellness.

Your Diet, Your Health

As I demonstrated in this book, the old cliché that "you are what you eat" has some truth to it. Our diets have a significant impact on our overall health. While foods that cause chronic inflammation in our bodies lead to more pain, foods that are rich in minerals have the power to prevent pain, illness, and the common maladies of aging. Quality supplements can likewise play a vital role in boosting our state of health.

Many diseases are caused or made worse by what we bring into our bodies. Neglecting nutrition and hydration create deficiencies in the body's natural levels of health. Excesses of toxins and unhealthy inflammatory foods create an environment for disease to develop and spread. The choices we make about our food, our water, our supplements, and even the packaging that all of these things come in are important and essential to our health. Correcting our diets to create the proper balance will restore the health and homeostasis we need to get better.

Making the right changes isn't always easy. Remaining set in our bad nutrition habits is the body's biggest obstacle to health. Nevertheless, you have the power to overcome this hurdle, and you have already taken the first step: by reading this book, you have given yourself the knowledge you need to set off on that road to recovery. Simply understanding which aspects of your eating habits need improvement is the foundation you need to develop your personal wellness diet.

When you give your body the proper nutrition, you give it the power to heal.

Whether you are combating a disease or simply seeking out a higher plateau of wellness, the following resources will help you achieve your healthy diet goals.

The End of All Disease

The Healthy Back Institute's website contains a wealth of information on how to use a good diet to maintain your health. Here you will find the latest news, breakthroughs, myth-busting secrets, and time-tested truths when it comes to healing yourself through the food you eat, the liquids you drink, and the supplements you take.

For access to the best information on nutritional supplements that will help your body heal and keep it healthy, visit www.endofalldiseases.com/supplementation. This page offers a wealth of supplement reviews and tips on how to leverage your supplements most effectively.

In my quest to find the best supplements for pain and inflammation, the products available on the market fell short of expectations. For that reason, the Healthy Back Institute spent years developing its own supplements, all of which take into account the knowledge, science, and philosophies of true healing detailed in this book. More information about these breakthrough supplements can be found at www.livingwellnutraceuticals.com.

Additionally, in my years as editor-in-chief of *Live Pain Free*, I have interviewed hundreds of experts about various aspects of diet, fitness, medicine, and health. You can access the best of these groundbreaking and enlightening interviews when you become a member of my *Live Pain Free* family, where you'll hear from experts like Dr. Jessica Black, Dr. Joel Fuhrman, Sally Fallon Morell, and other industry pioneers. Learn more at www.losethebackpain.com/membership.

Your Body, Your Health

It's no surprise that what we do with our bodies—not to mention what invades our bodies even when we least expect it—has a direct impact on how we feel physically.

You now know how you can make changes in your body to create a more positive outlook for your health, whether through addressing muscle imbalances and trigger points, improving circulation, or eliminating toxins and parasites. This is "self-health" at its best, and when you use the complete healing formula, the outcome really is in your hands.

While it isn't the only factor, your physical body is a critical part of the mind-body-diet Complete Healing Formula™. Treating the causes within your body through the approaches outlined in this book will lead you to the better health you want, and the rich way of life you deserve.

Because the body is the first (and usually the only) part of the mind-body-diet connection the modern medical establishment treats, there's no shortage of information on the topic at your disposal. However, in your quest for health, be sure to keep two things in mind. First, your body is just one part of the puzzle, and can't be addressed in isolation. Second, don't accept a treatment that only addresses your physical symptoms. Keep digging for the source of the problem so that you can achieve lasting wellness.

I can't stress enough how important it is to be informed about the real causes of your pain or illness. With so much misinformation on the market, researching the true root of the problem can be overwhelming. You've got to find sources of health information that aren't funded by pharmaceutical companies and that don't rely on selling ads or commercial airtime.

I stand behind the following health sources with my full trust and guarantee. To get regular news, tips, and condition-specific information online, visit these websites regularly:

- www.losethebackpain.com
- www.livepainfree.com
- www.endarthritisnow.com

You can also stay current on the latest breakthroughs in pain, health, and wellness by joining the *Live Pain Free* family. With membership in this community, you'll receive monthly newsletters, a CD each month featuring groundbreaking interviews with health experts like the ones you've read about in this book, access to exclusive one-on-one time with me, and much more. It's the best investment you can make in your health and wellness. To learn more, visit www.losethebackpain.com/membership.

Your Mind, Your Health

I hope I've thoroughly debunked the myth that our minds are disconnected from our health. My in-depth review of how our mental outlook, stress, and happiness can have an impact on how our bodies react to the environment should leave you with no doubt in the matter. I've given you the tools to take control of your emotional state and bring your body and mind into alignment—a union that will ultimately improve your overall health.

Our minds are intricately connected to the health of our bodies. Your emotional health has a tremendous impact on your physical health, and your state of mind has the power to either exacerbate your pain and illness or help you climb back to a level of health that will allow you to embrace life to the fullest again.

Beyond the information I've already given you in this book, I've compiled a list of resources to help you take your emotional balance to the next level to help you bring yourself closer to the true wellness you deserve. You can locate the Healthy Back Institute's expansive online resources on this subject for free, and we add to them all the time. Visit www.endofalldieases.com/healthy-mind for the complete list.

I've also spent time speaking with experts on the mind-health connection, and these discussions are included in my archives for my *Live Pain Free* members to enjoy. Learn more about this rewarding program, where you'll access more than five years' worth of groundbreaking mind, body, and diet healing tips at www.losethebackpain.com/membership.

All three areas of the Complete Healing Formula™—mind, body, and diet— are critical to your relief from pain and disease, as well as the level of health you enjoy overall. Now it's time to take what you've learned and embark on your own journey of discovery and self-healing.

Additional Ailment Solutions

I've given you a wealth of information on the true causes of and solutions for various ailments in the previous chapters. But the pages of any book are limited, and more resources and support are available for migraines, arthritis, chronic back pain, osteoporosis, fibromyalgia, heart disease, and cancer from the following sources:

Migraines

Additional tips, news, support, and migraine-related posts are available anytime at www.endofalldiseases.com/migraineresources. Or if you are suffering and haven't yet found a solution that works for you, you can contact us directly at the Healthy Back Institute. We are committed to giving you the guidance you need to find your way to a headache-free life.

Arthritis

I cited the work of Dr. Mark Wiley throughout these chapters, and he has literally written the book on the subject of arthritis. You can get a free copy of *Arthritis Reversed* at www.arthritisbookfree.com; just pay shipping costs. Dr. Wiley's book contains more in-depth information about arthritis, along with a thirty-day action plan to put a stop to this condition and regenerate your joints. If you're suffering from arthritis, this is a must-have resource on your journey to relief.

You can also get the joint support you need with what I consider to be the best joint supplement on the market. Endorsed not only by the Healthy Back Institute and *Live Pain Free*, Dr. Robert Thompson and thousands of customers also stand behind this supplement. Learn more about Super Joint Support ™ at www.losethebackpain.com/superjointsupport.html.

Chronic Back Pain

The Healthy Back Institute offers an endless supply of resources to help you eliminate chronic back pain from your life once and for all. Access my extensive knowledge about back pain by signing up for the *Live Pain Free* newsletter at www.losethebackpain.com/membership.

You can also access the Healthy Back Institute's full Lose the Back Pain® System™ and our safe and effective pain-relief products via our website. Visit the following links for more details:

- www.losethebackpain.com/101backpainrelieftips-warm3.html
- www.losethebackpain.com/7daybackpaincure.html
- www.losethebackpain.com/getstarted.html
- www.losethebackpain.com/inflammation5.html
- www.losethebackpain.com/rubonrelief.html

Osteoporosis

For more information about putting an end to osteoporosis once and for all, I highly recommend *The Calcium Lie* and *The Calcium Lie II*, by Dr. Robert Thompson. You can access a copy of Dr. Thompson's book at www.calciumliebook.com.

You can also get more osteoporosis support at www.losethebackpain.com/lpf-bones.html.

If you do nothing else for your health in this area, there's one thing I can't stress enough. Stop taking calcium supplements until you know for certain that you need them—and make sure you're getting all the other minerals you need to support true bone health.

Fibromyalgia

As one of the most nebulous and misunderstood conditions I've covered, it's difficult to give a single set of recommendations for fibromyalgia. But I've given you more than enough tools to begin your quest for healing in the preceding chapters. Additionally, I've compiled more resources about how you can eradicate fibromyalgia pain from your body and bring exuberance and vitality back into your life. You can access more information at www.endofalldiseases.com/fibroanswers.

Heart Disease

Heart disease is the number one cause of death in the United States. If you or someone you love is suffering from heart disease, you don't have to face it alone. A wealth of additional information is available to you in the Healthy Back Institute's 4-CD set, including *The Heart Disease Hoax*, available at www.losethebackpain.com/lpf-bones.

Cancer

As the second-biggest cause of death in the nation, cancer is getting a lot of attention right now. Not all the information out there is correct. I am always on the hunt for new cancer cures, and have several recent features and interviews available to my *Live Pain Free* members. Learn more at www.losethebackpain.com/membership.

A Future of Wellness

The time to take control of your health is now. Remember, to return your body and mind to a state of true wellness, action is key. You can read every book under the sun, but books are only as useful as your willingness to apply what you've read to your day-to-day life after the last page has been turned.

Use what I've shared with you in these pages about the Wellness Model of Health™ to make a fresh start with your body, mind, and diet. Take the first steps down the path to health and pain-free living. Give yourself permission to feel pain so that you can understand why it's happening and end it completely. Try new things, and trust that you will begin to feel better.

Literally tens of thousands of people have used the information in this book to drive pain and illness out of their lives forever. There is no reason why you can't do the same. Your return to health requires a commitment from you to apply focused, consistent action to the challenges ahead. Once you make that commitment, you will never go back to helplessness and suffering. Your life is your own, and so is your health.

A future of wellness is within your reach.

RECOMMENDED PRODUCTS

Heal-n-Soothe®

Heal-n-Soothe® combines the most powerful natural anti-inflammatory and pain-relieving ingredients known to man that have been scientifically proven to work. Plus, unlike non-steroidal anti-inflammatory drugs (NSAIDs), Heal-n-Soothe® has no dangerous side effects. This powerful pain-reliever was even referred to by one user as "God in a bottle."

www.healnsoothe.com

Rub on Relief®

Rub on Relief® is the *only* 100 percent all-natural topical pain cream designed to relieve *every* type of pain your body throws at you—and help you heal at the same time. This advanced topical analgesic anti-inflammatory cream delivers fast, penetrating pain relief of sore muscles and joints associated with arthritis, backache, strains, sprains, or any other type of pain.

www.rubonrelief.com

Super Joint Support™

Super Joint Support™ combines a unique, synergistic blend of cartilage-building, joint-lubricating, pain-relieving ingredients that deliver unprecedented relief. If you suffer from arthritis or osteoporosis, or fear they're in your future, this is a must-have supplement to protect your bones and joints.

www.superjointrelief.com

Lose the Back Pain® System™

Get rid of your back pain for good. Join over 175,000 people who have erased back pain from their lives. The Lose the Back Pain® System™ gives you the tools you need to assess the real cause of your pain, along with simple steps to treat and cure the pain yourself.

www.losethebackpain.com/getstarted

Lose the Neck Pain® System

Get rid of your neck pain once and for all with the Lose the Neck Pain® System. Developed after the monumental success of the Lose the Back Pain System, here you'll find the treatment and relief you need for your persistent neck and shoulder pain.

www.losetheneckpain.com

Healthy Back Institute's Premium Inversion Table

Undo the damage gravity has done to your entire body. Inversion therapy has been proven to reduce or eliminate various types of back and neck pain, not to mention improve circulation and brain function. With a money-back guarantee and backing from the Healthy Back Institute, there's no reason not to try inversion therapy.

www.tryinversion.com

Far Infrared Heating Pad

Harness the healing power of the sun's rays in the comfort of your bed, recliner, or car. This twenty-first century heating pad offers the ultimate in deep, penetrating heat relief. Your pain will melt away as the penetrating heat delivers more oxygen-rich blood to painful areas and speeds up your body's natural healing process.

www.farinfraredheatingpads.com

ElectroCleanse®

Begin ridding your body of parasites with this small-yet-effective device. The ElectroCleanse® uses precise electrical frequencies to exterminate harmful parasites from your body—parasites that are wreaking havoc on your health. Developed with the Dr. Clark Research Association, this tool is crucial to harnessing the healing of many major medical disorders.

www.losethebackpain.com/productreviews/electrocleanse.html

Sleepzyme®

Sleep soundly with the help of Mother Nature's ten most powerful sleep aids, all combined in Sleepzyme®. Effective sleep allows your body to heal itself while you rest and is a key to feeling more relaxed. This supplement is a must-have for anyone who feels stressed, tired, or simply wants to fall asleep faster and stay asleep longer.

www.natural-sleep-solution.com

Take Back Your Health Today

Maverick "Pioneer of Pain Relief" Shocks Medical Establishment - Again!

I'm opening up all my files and giving you access to all my research:

- **ALL** of the hidden, forgotten, and suppressed pain cures I've found

- **FULL** access to exclusive interviews with the world's most cutting-edge health experts

- **INCREDIBLE** stories of awe-inspiring healing directly from members just like you

- DVDs, CDs, access to a treasure trove of archives, new and exciting bonus material, and product reviews so you can discover what **REALLY** works for relieving pain

When you become a member of the family, you'll take control of your entire life!

The information, special savings, and direct access to my team of experts virtually ensures you'll start to feel better right away. Plus, with this vast knowledge bank of cutting-edge tips, you're going to not just live your life, but enjoy your life even more.

We live in exciting times. Just a few decades ago, we believed you either took a drug or got surgery for any illness, or that you were just stuck with what you got.

Today we know better.

You have more freedom of choice than you ever dreamed of.

You can give your body the right solutions to heal once and for all when you become a part of the Live Pain Free family.

As a reader of this book, I'm giving you four CDs, absolutely free, when you try my membership program today:

- Audio CD #1: How to Reverse Osteoporosis Naturally, with Vivian Goldschmidt, MA

- Audio CD #2: Once Illegal, Now FDA Approved: The Little-Known Treatment That Reverses Pain in Minutes, with Dr. Carol McMakin

- Audio CD #3: The Calcium Lie: What Your Doctor Doesn't Know Could Kill You, with Dr. Robert Thompson

- Audio CD #4: The Heart Disease Hoax: What Really Causes Heart Disease and How to Prevent and Reverse It, with Dr. Lundell

Plus, you'll have access to more than five years of interviews, special reports, newsletters, and more. Give yourself a break and try Live Pain Free today.

Visit: www.losethebackpain.com/membership